SPORT FIRST AID

UPDATED EDITION

Melinda J. Flegel, MS, ATC/R, CSCS

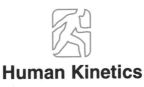

Human Kinetics

Library of Congress Cataloging-in-Publication Data

Flegel, Melinda J., 1958-
   Sport first aid / Melinda J. Flegel. -- Updated ed.
      p.   cm.
   "A publication for the American Sport Education Program and the
National Federation of State High School Associations."
   Includes bibliographical references and index.
   ISBN 0-88011-556-4
   1. Sports injuries.   2. First aid in illness and injury.
  I. Title.
  RD97.F525   1997
  617.1'0262--dc20

                                            96-22584
                                              CIP

ISBN: 0-88011-556-4

Acquisitions Editor: Jim Kestner; **Developmental Editor:** Jessie Daw; **Assistant Editors:** Lynn M. Hooper, Sandra Merz Bott, and Coree Schutter; **Copyeditor:** Barbara Walsh; **Indexer:** Theresa J. Schaefer; **Text Designer:** Keith Blomberg; **Graphic Artists:** Denise Lowry, Julie Overholt, Angie Snyder, Tara Welsch, and Yvonne Winsor; **Cover Designer:** Jack Davis; **Photographer (cover):** Wilmer Zehr; **Illustrator:** Tim Offenstein; **Printer:** United Graphics

Printed in the United States of America   10 9 8 7 6 5 4 3 2 1

Human Kinetics
Web site: http://www.humankinetics.com/

United States: Human Kinetics, P.O. Box 5076, Champaign, IL 61825-5076
1-800-747-4457
e-mail: humank@hkusa.com

Canada: Human Kinetics, Box 24040, Windsor, ON N8Y 4Y9
1-800-465-7301 (in Canada only)
e-mail: humank@hkcanada.com

Europe: Human Kinetics, P.O. Box IW14, Leeds LS16 6TR, United Kingdom
(44) 1132 781708
e-mail: humank@hkeurope.com

Australia: Human Kinetics, 57A Price Avenue, Lower Mitcham, South Australia 5062
(08) 277 1555
e-mail: humank@hkaustralia.com

New Zealand: Human Kinetics, P.O. Box 105-231, Auckland 1
(09) 523 3462
e-mail: humank@hknewz.com

Lord . . . all that we have accomplished you
have done for us.

Isaiah 26:12

Contents

Acknowledgments

I'd like to extend a special thanks to everyone who participated in the development of this updated edition: my colleague and friend Susan Kundrat for providing updated sports nutrition information; editors Jim Kestner, Lynn Hooper, and Jessie Daw for their support, patience, and extra effort in developmental editing; Rainer and Julie Martens and the rest of the Human Kinetics gang who made the production and distribution of this book possible; the expert reviewers for offering valuable suggestions for improving the book; and my family, friends, and co-workers for their never-ending support and encouragement.

Last but not least, I want to thank you, the reader, for your dedication to safety in sport and exercise.

Preface

Being a successful coach requires knowing more than just the skills and strategies of a sport. It includes being able to teach those techniques and tactics, motivate athletes, and manage a myriad of details. *And* it involves fulfilling the often forgotten role of being a competent first responder to players' injuries.

More than 5.25 million high school students participate in sports each year. The National Athletic Trainers' Association (NATA, 1989b) projects that more than one in five of these student-athletes—nearly 1.3 million—are injured annually. The majority of these injuries (62%) occur during practice, when medical personnel such as physicians and athletic trainers usually are not present. Consequently, as the coach, you are most often responsible for administering first aid to your injured athletes.

To help you meet this challenge, The American Sport Education Program (ASEP) has developed the Sport First Aid Course. This updated edition of the original *Sport First Aid* book serves as the text for that course.

The Sport First Aid Course, the widely used Coaching Principles Course, and the recently released Drugs and Sport Course comprise ASEP's Leader Level curriculum (see Appendix A).

Through a cooperative effort between ASEP and the National Federation of State High School Associations, ASEP is also the official education program for the National Federation Interscholastic Coaches Association. These three courses are known as the National Federation Interscholastic Coaches Education Program (NFICEP), and are delivered to interscholastic coaches throughout the nation.

Throughout its development and revision, this book was reviewed by a panel of experts representing each area of sports medicine specialization. Their close scrutiny and invaluable feedback ensure that this is a scientifically sound, relevant, and current text for coaches.

Specifically, *Sport First Aid* and its accompanying *Study Guide* are designed to help you do the following:

1. Develop a basic knowledge of sport injuries
2. Recognize common sport injuries
3. Administer appropriate sport first aid

ASEP hopes that by learning basic first aid skills for the sport setting, coaches like you will be better first responders to injured athletes. This is an excellent opportunity for you to expand your coaching skills. Moreover, it's a significant step toward providing a safer and more enjoyable sport experience for your athletes.

Learning Sport First Aid

Coach Mike Anderson is conducting a smooth-running midseason football practice on a cold and damp October day. Suddenly, after one scrimmage play, he hears a cry coming from the pile of players. As Coach Anderson helps the players unpile, he finds a groaning Kevin Green on the bottom of the stack. When asked what hurts, the second-string lineman moans, "My back, my back." Coach Anderson is not sure how bad the injury is because Kevin frequently has complained of injury in the past, sometimes feigning injury to avoid practice. Not knowing what to do, the coach takes no action, and Kevin eventually struggles to his feet. After practice, the athlete goes to a doctor who diagnoses the injury as a severe back sprain. Kevin is sidelined for the rest of the season.

Coaches with little understanding of first aid frequently choose the "do-nothing-until-I-have-to" option. Why? Primarily because they don't feel competent in offering first aid care. Unfortunately, this scenario is all too common. Studies have found that only about half the coaches nationwide are trained in either first aid or CPR (Rowe & Robertson, 1986; Weidner, 1989).

So what's the big deal? Any delay in first aid care can cause further injury or prolong an athlete's recovery time. Legwold (1983) reported that athletes who attended schools which did not employ a certified athletic trainer suffered a 71% reinjury rate, while those attending schools with a certified staff athletic trainer had only a 3% reinjury rate.

Then why not rely solely upon a certified athletic trainer to provide first aid care for athletes? First of all, only about 19% of high schools nationwide employ or contract a certified athletic trainer (Curtis, 1996). Secondly, it is nearly impossible for one athletic trainer to attend every practice and competition for a school's entire athletic program.

Realistically, then, coaches are relegated to the role of first responder to an athlete's injury. This responsibility requires a command of sport first aid knowledge and skills.

The American Sport Education Program (ASEP) believes that all coaches should be required to successfully complete training in both sport first aid and CPR. The reason? Athletes deserve competent care in emergencies that an untrained coach simply cannot provide.

ASEP wants to emphasize that this is a *sport first aid* book, not a general guide to anatomical sites and medical procedures. The word *sport* in the title reflects that the contents of this text are tailored to the athletic context. *First* refers to the coach's role as the initial responder to most athletes' injuries. And *aid* describes the help a coach properly trained in emergency care procedures can provide injured athletes. In other words, *Sport First Aid* encompasses the basic knowledge and skills needed to recognize sport-related injuries, provide appropriate emergency treatment, and ensure proper follow-up medical care. It specifically involves the recognition and emergency treatment of sport injuries on the playing field. Most basically, it entails learning what you should do and what you should *not* do when an athlete suffers an injury.

Sport first aid does not promote diagnosis and treatment by coaches. However, it does require coaches to make sure that injured athletes are seen and released by a physician before they return to action. And it includes these important tasks: contacting parents to inform them of the injury, calling emergency personnel to transport the injured athlete if necessary, assisting in safely moving the injured athlete to medical facilities, and encouraging an athlete during the rehabilitation process.

Part I of this text introduces you to the teamwork and preparation needed for effective sport first aid. In chapter 1 of this text you will learn your role as a coach on the sports medicine team. You will also learn how others will expect you to fulfill that role. Specifically, the text addresses parental and legal expectations. You'll meet the personnel with whom you'll be working, such as physicians, emergency medical technicians, physical therapists, and athletic trainers. Along with you, they make up the sports medicine team. In chapter 2, you will find out how to help prevent sport injuries. By training yourself in sport first aid and CPR, by conditioning athletes for competition, by fitting athletes with appropriate protective equipment, by enforcing correct sport technique and safety rules during practice and games, and by keeping playing areas free of safety hazards, you can provide the safest sporting environment possible.

In Part II you will learn the fundamentals of sport first aid. This includes increasing your knowledge of basic anatomy and sport first aid terminology covered in chapter 3. Chapter 4 will explain how to perform quick and accurate assessments of athletic injuries. With these general evaluation guidelines, you'll be prepared to learn how to provide basic emergency care procedures, described in chapter 5. Chapter 6 shows you how to safely move an injured athlete when necessary. These fundamentals are the essential foundation on which you can build your skills as a sport first aider.

In Part III you will learn the specific skills for responding to various sport injuries. Although chapters 7 through 11 cover less common injuries and illnesses, they are nonetheless important. Serious conditions such as circulatory and respiratory problems, head and spine injuries, internal organ injuries, sudden illness, and temperature-related illnesses are examined in these chapters. These problems do not occur often, but when they do, you'll want to be prepared to provide quick and appropriate first aid, perhaps to save an athlete's life. In chapters 12 through 14 you'll learn how to recognize and administer first aid for more common sport-related musculoskeletal problems, facial injuries, and skin conditions. You're likely to use these skills on a weekly—perhaps even daily—basis.

ASEP and the National Federation Interscholastic Coaches Association—through its National Federation Interscholastic Coaches Education Program (NFICEP)—originally developed this book as the text for their ASEP/NFICEP Sport First Aid Course, designed to provide interscholastic and club sport coaches with skills and a basic understanding of sports injuries. The course includes clinic, self-study, and testing phases. This text and the *Sport First Aid Study Guide* serve as primary resources for the course. Coaches who attend the Sport First Aid Clinic will learn emergency care skills and information through lecture and hands-on practice sessions. After the clinic, coaches must complete the exercises in the *Study Guide* and pass a written take-home test in order to receive recognition for successfully completing the course. For more information or to find out when the next Sport First Aid Course will be offered near you, contact ASEP by phone (800-747-5698) or e-mail (asep@hkusa.com), or check the calendar at ASEP's web site (http://www.asep.com/).

Armed with the information and skills from this *Sport First Aid* text and course, you will, ASEP hopes, be able to confidently and competently administer first aid to your athletes. The health and success of your athletes depend on it.

PART I

Introduction to Sport First Aid

Being a contributing member of a successful team requires teamwork and preparation. No athlete can walk onto a playing field and expect to contribute toward a victory if he or she is out of shape and unfamiliar with his or her teammates. Being an effective sport first aider is no different.

You must know not only your responsibilities and limitations, but also those of other members of the sports medicine team. Chapter 1 introduces you to your role as a player on the sports medicine team. You'll learn what parents and the legal authorities expect from you as a sport first aid provider. And you will become familiar with other members of the sports medicine team so you will know how to interact with them to make your efforts successful.

Just as an athlete needs preseason preparation or conditioning to achieve success, you also need to be prepared for your first aid duties. Chapter 2 will help you prepare preventive strategies to minimize injuries suffered by your athletes. These strategies include developing preseason conditioning programs, ensuring a safe playing environment, formulating an emergency plan, and enforcing proper sport skills and safety rules. Using these strategies, you can greatly reduce your athletes' risk of injury.

CHAPTER 1

Your Role as a Coach

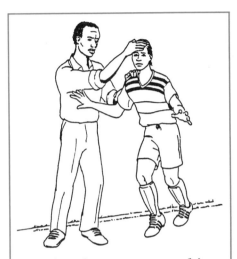

Imagine that you are coaching a high school soccer team. It's an incredibly hot and humid day, and your star forward staggers off the field. As you grab the player's arm and help him to the bench, you notice that his skin feels dry and very hot. You attempt to ask him questions, but he responds with incoherent mumbling. What's wrong with him? He has a flushed appearance, so could he be suffering from heatstroke? Some of the other players say that he is a diabetic. So is the athlete suffering from a heat or a diabetic illness? If the problem is related to diabetes, is it hyperglycemia or insulin shock, and how do you handle it? If you wait too long or treat the condition improperly, the athlete could die.

Recent studies have shown relatively high injury rates among high school athletes. Based on research conducted by the National Athletic Trainers' Association (NATA, 1989a, 1989b) from 1986 through 1989, an estimated 1.3 million U.S. high school athletes are injured each year. This means that more than 1 out of 5 high school athletes may require sport first aid. Another injury surveillance study conducted from 1979 to 1992, in which nearly 60,000 athletes in 20 high schools were monitored (Rice, 1995), found an injury rate of 30.6 per 100 athletes per season.

Table 1.1 shows a breakdown in the number of injuries for each sport that have been found during various research studies.

Table 1.1   Injury Rates for Various High School Sports

Sport	Injury rate/sport	Source
Basketball (boys and girls)	22.0%	(NATA, 1989b)
Basketball (boys)	29.2%	(Rice, 1995)
Basketball (girls)	34.5%	(Rice, 1995)
Cross-country (boys)	38.7%	(Rice, 1995)
Cross-country (girls)	61.4%	(Rice, 1995)
Football	36.0%	(NATA, 1989a)
Football	58.8%	(Rice, 1995)
Gymnastics (girls)	38.9%	(Rice, 1995)
Soccer (boys)	36.4%	(Rice, 1995)
Soccer (girls)	43.7%	(Rice, 1995)
Wrestling	27.0%	(NATA, 1989b)
Wrestling	49.7%	(Rice, 1995)

Now if you're thinking, "Wait a minute. No one ever said anything about caring for injuries when I agreed to coach," you're probably right. What they should have told you is that the first day you put that whistle around your neck, you indirectly agreed to be responsible for your athletes' health.

Expectations and Duties

Think about it. As coach, *you* are often the first person to see an injury. Because there is usually no medical personnel around, *you* are responsible for administering first aid care. Also, *you* have to decide whether an injured athlete can return to play or should be sent to get medical help. Certainly, if your team or school is assisted by an athletic trainer or team physician, you should seek their advice; but it's unlikely that those personnel will be present for every practice or game.

Athletes typically look to their coaches for all the answers. However, parents, legal authorities, and other players on the sports medicine team also have certain expectations of coaches. Your role as a sport first aider is shaped by all these expectations.

Parents' Expectations

Parents will look to you for direction when their children are injured. They may ask questions like these:

> *What do you think is wrong with my daughter's knee?*
>
> *Will it get worse if she continues playing?*
>
> *Should she see a doctor?*
>
> *Does my son need to wear protective knee braces for football?*
>
> *What kind of taping can you do to prevent my son from reinjuring his ankle?*
>
> *When can he start competing again?*

And it's not enough to simply respond, "I don't know." You must either have the answer or, more likely, know how to get the answer quickly. Parents won't accept anything less.

Legal Authorities' Expectations

Gymnast Kim Evans flew off the uneven bars one day and crashed to the floor. Because she was lying facedown and appeared to be unconscious, Coach Sue Calhoun rolled her over to make sure she was breathing. Kim had sustained a back fracture and

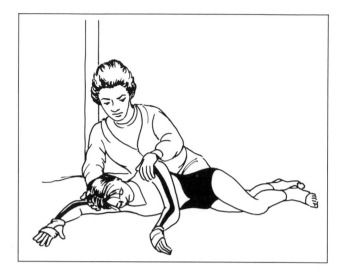

lost the function of both legs. Sue Calhoun was sued by Kim's parents and found negligent for failing to provide appropriate emergency medical assistance.

Unfortunately, with sports comes the risk of injury; sometimes, very serious injury. But if Coach Calhoun had had adequate preparation and practice in sport first aid, it's possible that Kim's back injury would not have caused nerve damage. And, in the end, Coach Calhoun would not have been found negligent.

Don't let the threat of lawsuits interfere with your learning sport first aid and utilizing it to help your athletes. All you have to do is follow nine simple legal duties (Martens, 1997).

Nine Legal Duties of a Coach

1. Properly plan the activity.
   - Make sure that athletes are in proper condition.
   - Teach athletes the sport skills in a progression so that they are adequately prepared to handle more difficult skills.
2. Provide proper instruction.
   - Keep up to date on better and safer ways of performing sport techniques.
   - Teach athletes the rules and the correct skills and strategies of the sport.
3. Provide a safe physical environment.
   - Monitor current environmental conditions (i.e., wind chill, temperature, and humidity).
   - Periodically inspect playing areas, the locker room, the weight room, and the dugout for hazards.

- Remove all hazards.
- Prevent improper or unsupervised use of facilities.

4. Provide adequate and proper equipment.
   - Make sure athletes are using top-quality equipment.
   - Inspect the equipment regularly.
   - Teach athletes how to fit, use, and inspect their equipment.

5. Match your athletes.
   - Match athletes according to size, physical maturity, skill level, and experience.

6. Evaluate athletes for injury or incapacity.
   - Enforce rules requiring all athletes to submit to preseason physicals and screenings to detect potential health problems.
   - If an athlete is not able to compete without pain or loss of function (i.e., inability to walk, run, jump, throw, etc. without restriction), immediately remove her or him from the activity.

7. Supervise the activity closely.
   - Do not allow athletes to practice difficult or potentially dangerous skills without proper supervision.
   - Forbid horseplay.
   - Do not allow athletes to use sport facilities without supervision.

8. Warn of inherent risks.
   - Provide parents and athletes with both oral and written statements of the inherent health risks of their particular sport.

9. Provide appropriate emergency assistance.
   - Learn sport first aid.
   - Use only the skills that you are qualified to administer.

If you aren't already, become familiar with each of these legal duties. The first eight duties deal mainly with preventive measures, explained more thoroughly in chapter 2. Most of this book is designed to help you handle duty number 9.

The Ninth Legal Duty

The legal system has definite expectations in regard to duty number 9—providing appropriate emergency assistance. If an athlete is injured, you are legally expected to do the following:

- *Take Action When Needed*
  The law assumes that when you agreed to coach, you indirectly agreed to provide first aid care for any injury or illness suffered by any athlete under your supervision. Therefore, if no medical personnel are present when an injury occurs, you are responsible for providing emergency care.
- *Provide a Certain Standard of Care*
  If you give emergency care, you must use standard procedures. What are "standard" procedures? Most often, these are techniques taught in basic first aid and cardiopulmonary resuscitation (CPR) courses. To learn these standards, you should attend certification courses taught by the American Red Cross or the American Heart Association. If you have taken other courses or attended workshops on emergency medical procedures or athletic injury care, you will also be expected to provide the standard of care taught in those educational settings.

Some states expect coaches to meet additional standards of care. Check with your athletic director to find out if your state has specific guidelines for the quality of care to be provided by coaches.

Good Samaritan Law

Many coaches fail to fully appreciate their legal responsibilities; many others are so fearful of providing emergency medical care that they fail to act promptly in injury situations. Neither approach is adequate.

You cannot ignore the nine legal duties of coaching. Furthermore, you should not be afraid to take action when injuries occur. If you provide emergency care to the best of your ability, you may be protected by what is called the Good Samaritan law.

This law varies from state to state, so check with your athletic director or state coaches' association to make sure you are covered. Specifically, ask whether the Good Samaritan law protects you if, in good faith, you do the best you can in administering initial emergency care. And whether it does or doesn't, don't just stand on the sidelines.

Learn more about sport first aid so you will be a confident and competent first responder to your athletes' injuries.

Consent

Legally, you must have an adult's consent before you can give first aid care. For minors, obtain a signed written consent form from their parents before the season begins. For injured adult athletes, you should specifically ask them whether they want your help. If they are unconscious, consent is usually implied. If they refuse help, you are not required to provide it. In fact, if you still attempt to give care, they can sue you for assault.

So as you can see, the expectations of the legal community regarding coaches' emergency care behavior are quite high. You must be prepared to meet them. And a good place to start is by consulting the *Coaches Guide to Sport Law* (Nygaard & Boone, 1985), which you can obtain through ASEP.

Your Role on the Sports Medicine Team

As a coach, you are an important member of the sports medicine team. You can assist the sports medicine professionals by doing the following:

- Help to prevent injuries through the use of proper training methods, safe and effective sport technique instruction, and close and constant supervision.
- Prevent further harm to an injured athlete.
- Ensure that an injured athlete receives prompt medical attention.
- Provide information regarding an athlete's injury.
- Act as a liaison between emergency professionals and the injured athlete.
- Provide emergency care if a medical professional is unavailable.

To be a vital part of the team, you have to be familiar with your teammates—the health professionals who will assist you in caring for an injured athlete.

Emergency Medical Personnel

Emergency Medical Technicians (EMTs) and paramedics are specially trained to handle medical emergencies and serious injuries. They are highly skilled in evaluating and monitoring injuries and serious medical problems, as well as providing basic medical care. They are also very competent in immobilizing people with serious injuries and providing swift and safe transportation to emergency medical facilities.

You should try to become familiar with the emergency medical personnel in your area. These people are often willing to volunteer their time and rescue vehicles to provide emergency care during tournaments and contests involving contact sports such as football or wrestling.

Once the rescue squad arrives, let them take over the care of the athlete. Remember, they handle health emergencies every day and are better trained for doing so than you. Your role should be simply to assist them as needed. In that regard, be prepared to

1. take charge of crowd control,
2. assist in moving the athlete, and
3. provide information on how the injury occurred.

Unfortunately, EMTs are not always readily available. If emergency personnel are not present when an athlete is injured, your role is to

1. protect the athlete from further harm,
2. send someone to call emergency medical personnel, if necessary,
3. evaluate the injury,
4. administer first aid, and
5. provide information on how the injury occurred.

Physicians

The head coach of the sports medicine team is the physician. He or she alone is qualified to diagnose athletic injuries. Further, the physician is also the individual who should direct all treatment and rehabilitation of an injury and supervise the actions of other members of the team.

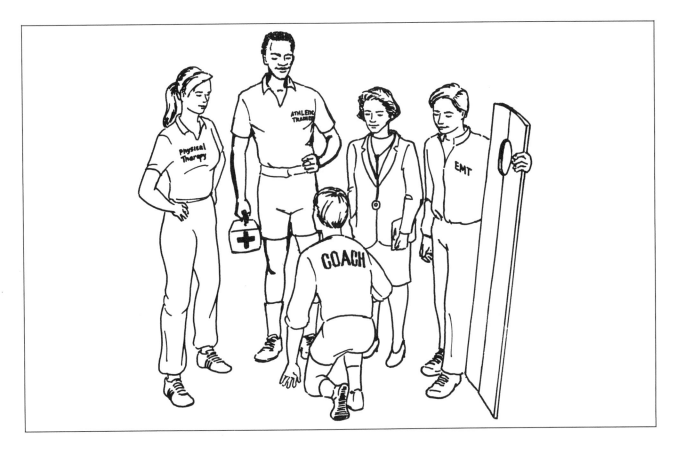

The question you might ask is this: Out of all the types of physicians available, which one should an injured athlete see—a family practitioner, pediatrician, orthopedist, podiatrist? The answer is ultimately up to the athlete's parents or legal guardian, but they may ask for your advice. To help you respond knowledgeably, here is a brief description of the common categories of sport physicians.

Types of Physicians

Although any physician can diagnose and direct the treatment of an injured athlete, a physician who specializes in sports medicine is a definite plus. These sports medicine specialists are sensitive to the special needs of athletes and will do all they can to get athletes back to full participation as quickly and as safely as possible.

Family practitioners specialize in general medicine for families. This includes infants all the way through to senior citizens.

Pediatricians specialize in providing medical care for children. This usually encompasses infants to teenagers.

Orthopedists are sometimes called bone doctors. Actually, they are trained in the clinical and surgical care of injuries to the bones, muscles, and other joint tissues such as cartilage, tendons, and ligaments.

Podiatrists, or foot doctors, provide medical and surgical care for leg and foot problems only. They also make special support inserts for shoes to correct alignment problems of the feet and legs.

Many of the physician specialty groups, such as orthopedics and pediatrics, offer special sports medicine training courses to their members. When seeking specific care for an injured athlete, you may want to find a particular physician who has sports medicine training within his or her field of specialization. Check the yellow pages of your phone book under "Physicians" and look for those that list services in sports medicine. Physician costs will vary depending on the services rendered and whether X rays are taken.

If you cannot find a physician with sports medicine training, then a physician who is personally active in sports and exercise may be a good alternative. Such a physician is also likely to be sensitive to an injured athlete's unique needs.

As a coach, you should attempt to establish a close working relationship with a physician. You may ask for his or her assistance in conducting team physicals or in teaching sports medicine basics to your coaching staff. Many physicians volunteer their time to provide medical coverage for home games. They may also offer to assist you with preseason physicals and screenings.

Once an athlete has been examined by a physician, it's important that you support the physician's recommendations. This includes following any restrictions on an athlete's playing time. If the parent or legal guardian is not satisfied with the physician's diagnosis and treatment, seeking a second opinion may be warranted. However, it is unethical for either the parents/guardians or you to send an athlete to a different physician in an attempt to get permission for the athlete to resume activity.

Physical Therapists (PTs)

Physical therapists are licensed health professionals who rehabilitate individuals suffering from disease or injury. They are trained to analyze a patient's strength, joint motion, coordination, and other physical attributes and then instruct the patient in an individualized rehabilitation program. Therapists are also trained in administering modalities such as whirlpools, massage, ultrasound, muscle stimulation, and manipulations to help ease pain, decrease swelling, and promote tissue healing.

Physical therapists, or PTs as they are often called, are trained to handle a wide variety of medical problems, including cerebral palsy, strokes, heart problems, paraplegia, and burns. PTs may also specialize in handling sport injuries. To do so, they must complete several years of clinical sports medicine experience and successfully pass a sport physical therapy examination. Such individuals are then recognized as sport physical therapists.

An athlete requiring the services of a physical therapist should check with a local sports medicine clinic, physical therapy clinic, or hospital physical therapy department or should obtain a referral by a physician. Physi-

---

For Sport Rehabilitation

DO NOT . . .

. . . change an athlete's rehabilitation program.

. . . try to decide when an athlete's rehabilitation is complete.

---

cian referral is not necessary in some states, however. The rehabilitation program that a physical therapist prescribes to an injured athlete can be crucial to the athlete's complete recovery.

You can also help by encouraging athletes to do their rehabilitation exercises.

The decision to alter or discontinue an athlete's rehabilitation program must be made by a qualified physical therapist. PTs can also help you evaluate your athletes' fitness components such as strength, flexibility, and coordination. And they can provide assistance as you screen and condition your athletes. Finally, physical therapists can offer you valuable tips on proper exercise technique for your athletes.

Certified Athletic Trainers (ATC)

Athletic trainers are nationally certified allied health professionals trained in the recognition, treatment, rehabilitation, and prevention of athletic injuries. They evaluate and provide immediate care for injuries on the playing field, court, and running track. ATCs also fit athletes with protective padding and equipment and provide supportive taping and protective bandaging. Athletic trainers must work under the supervision of a physician and most often work at high schools, colleges, and sports medicine or physical therapy centers.

If you work with an athletic trainer, it is her or his role to evaluate and care for an injured athlete. During practices and games, it is the trainer's responsibility to decide whether a recently injured athlete can resume playing or must rest. The trainer can also help to prevent injuries by screening athletes and developing and implementing preseason conditioning programs.

Sport First Aid Recap

1. You play a vital role on the sports medicine team, providing emergency care for injured athletes if medical personnel are not present.

2. Athletes and their parents expect you, as a coach, to be a competent first aid provider.

3. One of the nine legal duties of coaches is to provide appropriate medical assistance. The law requires you to act and to provide a standard of care commensurate with your training. You can be ruled negligent if you fail to do so.

4. You can be a big help to the health professionals who are qualified to care for injured athletes. At times, your biggest contribution will be providing information regarding how an injury occurred and encouraging the athlete during rehabilitation.

CHAPTER 2

Sport First Aid Game Plan

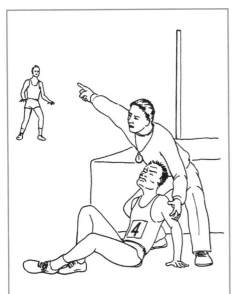

During preseason conditioning, high jumper Sean Morris hurts his knee while doing explosive plyometric power training. Coach Flint needs only to glance at the injury to notice an obvious deformity to Sean's knee. The coach can see that Sean is in a lot of pain, so he wants to get medical help as quickly as possible. He sends one of the other track athletes to call for help. After discovering that the coach's office is locked, the athlete returns to get Coach Flint's office keys, only to find the coach far from the high jump pit, searching frantically for a splint for Sean's leg. After several minutes, Coach Flint returns and gives the athlete his keys to the office. Sean is treated and transported by emergency medical personnel nearly an hour after he was hurt.

To get your team ready for games, you have to plan practices, develop playing strategies, and prepare your players. Through experience you know that this pregame planning process is essential to success. The same is true for sport first aid. To handle injuries effectively, you have to plan for them. But you cannot learn how to prepare for injuries through trial and error.

Indeed, your actions during the first few minutes of an injury are critical. There may be blood loss, swelling, breathing difficulties, and a whole host of other problems. If you act quickly and appropriately, you can minimize the damage created by the injury. Ultimately, this will help to speed an injured athlete's recovery.

So, to ensure that your sport first aid game plan is ready, read this chapter closely and use it to prepare. These are the key parts of the first aid strategy to make you an effective contributor:

- Learning sport first aid
- Keeping athletes' health records
- Checking facilities and equipment
- Getting players ready to perform
- Developing an emergency plan

Learning Sport First Aid

Much of our learning happens in progressive stages. So, to prepare you to assume your first aid responsibilities, this book will take you through a three-step learning process in which you

1. learn the basics of sport first aid,
2. learn how to recognize common sport injuries, and
3. learn how to provide appropriate first aid for these common injuries.

You also need to know how to prepare an injured athlete for transportation to medical facilities and how to contact appropriate medical personnel. This book and the ASEP/NFICEP Leader Level Sport First Aid Course will help you learn all these things and more.

However, ASEP strongly recommends that you supplement what you learn from this book and from the course with certification in basic first aid and cardiopulmonary resuscitation (CPR). The American Red Cross offers certification in both areas, while the American Heart Association offers CPR certification. The procedures taught in these programs are recognized nationally as standards for providing first aid care. If you become certified in either first aid or CPR, you will be expected to provide the standard of care taught in the certification program.

Every Coach Should Be Certified in CPR!

Keeping Current

Because so many improvements are constantly being made in sports medicine, you cannot just learn sport first aid once and think you're set for life. You can be certain that the sport first aid techniques used in the future will be much different and better than the methods advocated now. So keep yourself up to date with the latest in sport first aid by doing the following:

- Read current sports medicine books and articles to learn the newest techniques. Some excellent sources of information are listed in the Recommended Readings on page 175.
- Keep your first aid and CPR certifications current. First aid certifications generally expire after 3 years, whereas CPR cards must be renewed every year. Recertification is vital; it enables you to stay up on the latest first aid techniques.
- Attend sports medicine and sport first aid seminars and clinics. The ASEP/NFICEP Leader Level Sport First Aid Course will be updated as advances in this area warrant, so plan to attend another course in the next few years (see Appendix A).

Recognizing Limitations

Although you may educate yourself extensively in sport first aid, don't attempt the duties of a physician. Recognize your limitations. Don't try to give care unless you're qualified to do it. Also, if medical personnel are present, give them complete control to handle any injuries; assist them if they request it. The damage you can cause by overstepping the limits of your training may be suffered by an athlete for many years. And if you do act irresponsibly and harm an athlete, you will probably be the target of a lawsuit.

Keeping Athletes' Health Records

Like most coaches, you probably have statistical records of your team's game performances filed away in your office. But do you have a filing cabinet for players' health information? If not, get one. Then collect from each player these three items:

- Consent form
- Health history form
- Emergency information card

Consent Form

As we discussed in chapter 1 regarding legal duties, you cannot give first aid care to a minor unless you have consent. Before the season, you must have parents or legal guardians complete and return an explicitly worded consent form for their children. A form similar to the one shown in Figure 2.1 informs the parent(s) or guardian(s) of the inherent risks of sport and requests permission for the child to be treated for injury.

Health History Form

It is very important for you to know whether any of your athletes have health problems that could affect their sport participation. Diabetes, asthma, epilepsy, heart murmurs,

---

INFORMED CONSENT FORM

I hereby give my permission for _____ to participate in _____
during the athletic season beginning in _____. Further, I authorize the school to provide emergency treatment of any injury or illness my child may experience if qualified medical personnel consider treatment necessary and perform the treatment. This authorization is granted only if I cannot be reached and a reasonable effort has been made to do so.

Date _____ Parent or guardian _____

Address _____ Phone (____) _____

Family physician _____ Phone (____) _____

Medical conditions (e.g., allergies or chronic illnesses) _____

_____

Other person to contact in case of emergency: _____

Relationship with person _____ Phone (____) _____

My child and I are aware that participating in _____ is a potentially hazardous activity. I assume all risks associated with participation in this sport, including but not limited to falls, contact with other participants, the effects of the weather, traffic, and other reasonable risk conditions associated with the sport. All such risks to my child are known and appreciated by me.

I understand this informed consent form and agree to its conditions on behalf of my child.

Child's signature _____ Date _____

Parent's signature _____ Date _____

Figure 2.1 Informed consent form.

and skin conditions are some of the health problems you should know about. If a physician clears an athlete with a health problem for participation, you should have a record of the following:

1. The health problem
2. Special medications the athlete may need to take
3. Activity restrictions for the athlete

A health history form (see Figure 2.2) will give you this information.

Emergency Information Card

In the event of an emergency, you must be able to contact the athlete's parents or guardian and physician. An emergency information card (see Figure 2.3) will give you their names and numbers. It should also alert you to information on any preexisting medical

problems that may influence the treatment of an athlete.

This card must be completed by the athlete's parents before the season. In cases where you are practicing or playing away from your office, you will want to take a copy of the card.

Checking Facilities and Equipment

Although preparation and care of the playing area may be the responsibility of a groundskeeper or janitor, you are still responsible for checking its safety. Litter, slippery floors, broken goals, worn playing surfaces, and countless other problems can lead to injury. Be sure to check for any hazards and have them fixed before the season. See ASEP's

ATHLETIC MEDICAL EXAMINATION FOR _____
(Sport)

Name _____ Age _____ Birthdate _____ S.S.# _____

Address _____ Phone no. _____
(Street)　　　　　　　　　　(City)　　　　　　(Zip)

Instructions:

All questions must be answered. Failure to disclose pertinent medical information may invalidate your insurance coverage and may cancel your eligibility to participate in interscholastic athletics. Any further health problems must be discussed with the physician at the time of this examination.

Medical history:

Have you ever had any of the following? If "yes" give <u>details</u> to the examining doctor.

	No	Yes	Details (if yes)
1. Head injury or concussion			
2. Bone or joint disorders, fractures (broken bones), dislocations, trick joints, arthritis, back pain			
3. Eye or ear problems (disease or surgery)			
4. Dizzy spells, fainting, or convulsions			
5. Tuberculosis, asthma, bronchitis			
6. Heart trouble or rheumatic fever			
7. High or low blood pressure			
8. Anemia, leukemia, or bleeding disorder			
9. Diabetes, hepatitis, or jaundice			
10. Ulcers, other stomach trouble, or colitis			
11. Kidney or bladder problems			
12. Hernia (rupture)			
13. Mental illness or nervous breakdown			
14. Addiction to drugs or alcohol			
15. Surgery or advised to have surgery			
16. Taking medication regularly			
17. Allergies or skin problems			
18. Other illness, injury not named above			
19. Menstrual problems; LMP			

Signature _____

Date _____

Figure 2.2 Health history form.

EMERGENCY INFORMATION CARD

Athlete's name _____ Age _____

Address _____

Phone _____ S.S.# _____

Sport _____

List two persons to contact in case of emergency:

Parent or guardian's name _____ Home phone _____

Address _____ Work phone _____

Second person's name _____ Home phone _____

Address _____ Work phone _____

Relationship to athlete _____

Insurance co. _____ Policy no. _____

Physician's name _____ Phone _____

IMPORTANT

Are you allergic to any drugs? _____ If so, what? _____

Do you have any other allergies? (i.e., bee sting, dust) _____

Do you suffer from _____ asthma, _____ diabetes, or _____ epilepsy? (Check any that apply.)

Are you on any medication? _____ If so, what? _____

Do you wear contacts? _____

Other:

Signature _____ Date _____

Figure 2.3 Emergency information card.

Successful Coaching (Martens, 1997), pages 161-164, for a checklist.

Sports equipment also needs to be checked before the season. You must inspect sticks, rackets, bats, gymnastic apparatus, and other equipment for damage. And be sure that goalposts, net standards, landing pits, and gymnastic apparatus are well padded.

You'll also want to have some very valuable equipment on hand in case of injury. This will make up the first aid kit. You should have a first aid kit and ice cooler on the sidelines of every practice and game.

When preparing your first aid kit, omit all medicines, both over-the-counter and prescription drugs; it is illegal for you to give any kind of medicine to athletes. This includes aspirin or any other over-the-counter pain medicine.

Don't include iodine either. It may cause an allergic reaction in some individuals. Stock your kit only with those items necessary for administering basic sport first aid.

Getting Players Ready to Perform

Athletes who are not in shape are more likely to be injured. Yet, many coaches frequently neglect measures to ensure that every athlete is fit to play. You can get ahead of other coaches' programs by instituting these vital methods for preventing injuries:

- Preseason physical exam
- Preseason screening

- Preseason conditioning
- Proper warm-up and cool-down
- Protective equipment, bracing, and taping
- Correct skill instruction
- Sound nutritional guidance
- Ban on horseplay

Preseason Physical Exam

The first step in preparing an athlete for sport participation is to require a preseason physical. This should be a very thorough examination conducted by a physician.

During the physical the physician should perform a general health exam, as well as circulatory, respiratory, neurological, orthopedic, vision, and hearing examinations. The athlete should also undergo routine blood and urine analyses. The physician should note and consider any preexisting or potential health problems when deciding whether an athlete is cleared to participate.

All athletes must turn in their physical forms prior to the season. All forms should be kept on file for future reference.

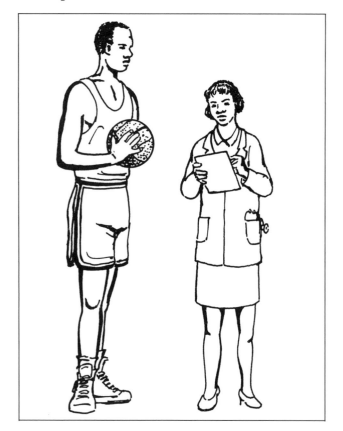

DISQUALIFYING MEDICAL CONDITIONS

Some common problems found by the examining physician that could disqualify athletes from competition or limit their participation include the following:

Diabetes
Asthma
Heart conditions
High blood pressure
Epilepsy
Previous head injuries
Previous spinal injuries
Chronic orthopedic problems (e.g.,unstable knees, ankles, shoulders)

Preseason Screening

Although the physical exam will detect specific health problems, it does not provide insight about an athlete's overall fitness. Coaches obtain this information through preseason screening.

Preseason screening should be conducted in the off-season by a specially trained health or fitness professional, such as a physical therapist or athletic trainer. Each athlete should be evaluated for the following:

- *Strength* in the muscle groups most often used in the particular sport—for example, a football player's neck strength or a basketball player's ankle strength
- *Flexibility* or tightness in the major muscle groups
- *Cardiovascular endurance* (especially for endurance athletes such as cross-country runners, track athletes, triathletes, and cyclists)
- *Body composition* or percent body fat (especially important for wrestlers, gymnasts, and track athletes who severely restrict their diets to control their weight)

These tests pinpoint potential fitness problems that can lead to injury. Coaches or athletic trainers should teach athletes conditioning exercises to help them improve any problems before the season.

Preseason Conditioning

Coaches should have athletes start a conditioning program before the season to get them in shape. The conditioning exercises focus on muscle strength, endurance, flexibility, power, and speed needed for the sport. To get in shape, athletes must begin working out at least 6 to 8 weeks before the season. It takes at least that long for athletes to achieve any improvements in these fitness attributes.

To improve strength, athletes need to perform at least three sets of 6 to 8 repetitions of each exercise, 3 days a week. Postpubescent athletes should lift at least 70% of their maximum to gain strength. With prepubescent athletes, to avoid weight lifting-related injuries, emphasize activities that require the athletes to support their own body weight (e.g., push-ups). Training 3 days a week for at least 20 continuous minutes is necessary to improve cardiovascular endurance. Also, athletes should perform stretching exercises at least 5 days a week.

These are just the most basic guidelines for training athletes. For more information on preseason screening and conditioning, consult ASEP's *Coaches Guide to Sport Physiology* (Sharkey, 1986).

Proper Warm-Up and Cool-Down

Be sure that your athletes warm up before their conditioning workouts, practices, and games. This doesn't mean going out 5 minutes before practice and hitting or throwing a few balls. A proper warm-up is an exercise routine that prepares the body for vigorous physical activity. Athletes should warm up at least 15 minutes prior to activity using this sequence:

1. *General body warm-up.* Have athletes jog or bike at a low intensity or perform light calisthenics for 5 to 10 minutes. The intensity of the general warm-up should cause a slight increase in the heart and breathing rates. It should also cause the athlete to break into a

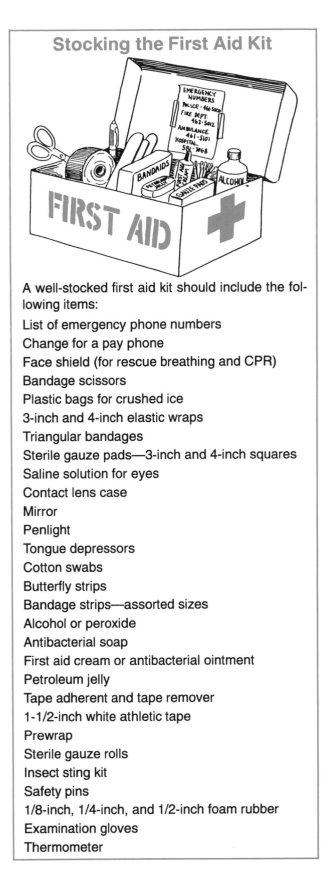

Stocking the First Aid Kit

A well-stocked first aid kit should include the following items:

List of emergency phone numbers
Change for a pay phone
Face shield (for rescue breathing and CPR)
Bandage scissors
Plastic bags for crushed ice
3-inch and 4-inch elastic wraps
Triangular bandages
Sterile gauze pads—3-inch and 4-inch squares
Saline solution for eyes
Contact lens case
Mirror
Penlight
Tongue depressors
Cotton swabs
Butterfly strips
Bandage strips—assorted sizes
Alcohol or peroxide
Antibacterial soap
First aid cream or antibacterial ointment
Petroleum jelly
Tape adherent and tape remover
1-1/2-inch white athletic tape
Prewrap
Sterile gauze rolls
Insect sting kit
Safety pins
1/8-inch, 1/4-inch, and 1/2-inch foam rubber
Examination gloves
Thermometer

light sweat. This helps to prepare the heart, lungs, muscles, and tendons for vigorous activity. Ultimately it helps to prevent injury as well as improve performance.

2. *Stretching exercises.* After a general warm-up, athletes should stretch the major muscles of the

- shoulders,
- arms and forearms,
- trunk (back and abdominal areas),
- thighs, and
- lower legs.

Each muscle group should be stretched in one or more repetitions for a total of 15 to 30 seconds during the warm-up. To prevent athletes from bouncing while stretching, you may want to make sure that they hold a stretch for at least 10 seconds. The purpose of warm-up stretching is to loosen up the muscles for activity (see Appendix B).

3. *Sport specific drills.* These are drills in which athletes practice the skills of the particular sport. For example, sport-specific softball drills include batting and throwing. In tennis and racquetball drills, players practice serves as well as backhand and forehand shots.

At the end of each practice, workout, game, meet, or match, athletes should gradually cool their bodies down. In other words, they should slowly reduce the intensity of their activity until their heart and breathing rates drop to near-normal resting levels. Suddenly stopping exercise inhibits one's recovery from activity and can lead to problems such as fainting. Athletes should perform cool-down activities such as walking or jogging for 5 to 10 minutes.

The cool-down should conclude with stretching. Since the muscles are very warm after activity, they will stretch more easily and maintain the stretched position longer. That's why the cool-down period is a prime time for athletes to achieve long-term improvements in their flexibility. Each muscle group should be stretched for a total of 2 to 3 minutes. In general, muscles need to be stretched for a total of 2 to 5 minutes a day to obtain lasting improvements in length. Stretches for each muscle group can be performed all at once or be broken down into repetitions performed throughout the day.

Protective Equipment, Bracing, and Taping

Every athlete needs to be instructed in the fitting and wearing of safety equipment for his or her particular sport. This is especially true in football, where helmets must be specially fitted and the athletes are required to wear all of their protective pads. You should be familiar with the protective equipment required for your sport and how to fit it properly.

Two often-neglected but important pieces of equipment are safety glasses or goggles, and mouthpieces. If there is any chance of eye injury, particularly in contact or racket sports, athletes must wear safety eyewear. Also, expensive dental repairs can be avoided if athletes in contact sports wear protective mouth guards.

What about protective bracing and taping? You may have heard about coaches who require certain football players to wear prophylactic knee braces or basketball players to tape their ankles, even though the athletes have not suffered previous injuries in these areas. The coaches feel that braces or tape will help prevent injury.

TO BRACE OR NOT TO BRACE?

Are protective bracing and taping all they're cracked up to be? They are certainly no substitute for being in shape. Remember that strength, flexibility, endurance, and power are the keys to preventing injury. Bracing and taping are of secondary importance. The results of studies investigating the effectiveness of protective bracing and taping are inconclusive. It is very difficult to prove whether a decrease in injuries can be attributed to wearing a protective brace. Ultimately the issue of preventive bracing and taping is decided by the individual preference and financial status of the athletic program and athlete.

Correct Skill Instruction

Many athletes are injured because they use incorrect technique. In football, since spear tackling with the head was ruled illegal, the number of head and neck injuries among players has decreased. Baseball or softball players who dive headfirst into the base instead of sliding feetfirst are prone to tooth, head, and neck injuries. Many tennis players suffer from tennis elbow because they use incorrect backhand techniques.

You can help prevent these and other injuries by simply teaching your athletes safe and proper performance techniques. And keep an eye out to correct athletes who use potentially harmful techniques. Warn them of the possible injuries they could suffer, then reinstruct them in the appropriate maneuvers.

Sound Nutritional Guidance

Encourage your athletes to eat balanced meals according to the food guide pyramid. Figure 2.4 outlines the components and amounts of each dietary source recommended for athletes.

Also encourage athletes to drink plenty of water all day long. Particularly important, athletes should drink 1 to 2 cups of water 30 minutes before exercise and 1/2 to 1 cup every 15 to 20 minutes during practices or games. For activities lasting over 60 minutes, athletes may benefit from a sport drink, which is generally a combination of a carbohydrate source, the electrolytes potassium and sodium, and water. A sport drink with the proper carbohydrate content of 6 to 7% (14-17 grams of carbohydrate per 240 ml) may enhance fluid absorption and provides continuous carbohydrates to working muscles.

For Hydration

DO NOT . . .

. . . give athletes salt tablets to prevent dehydration. Excess salt in the stomach actually pulls water into the stomach. This leaves less water to help cool the body through sweat.

Contrary to popular belief, athletes do not need to take vitamin, mineral, protein, or carbohydrate supplements. By eating a balanced diet, they will get all of the nutrients they need for competition.

Eating on the Road

An adequate, high-carbohydrate, moderate-protein, low-fat diet can be obtained on the road with a little planning and organization. If budgets allow, bring along dried fruits, juices, low-fat granola bars, and other snacks that offer healthy alternatives to vending machines. In addition, many restaurants will honor special requests for teams, such as pasta bars, low-fat sandwich options, and fresh fruits and vegetables. Encourage athletes to consume juices and skim milk products as opposed to soft drinks; baked, broiled, or boiled meats instead of fried meats; and plenty of carbohydrate-rich foods such as potatoes, rice, pasta, breads, bagels, fruits, and vegetables. Portions must be appropriate, and be sure to plan meals to allow

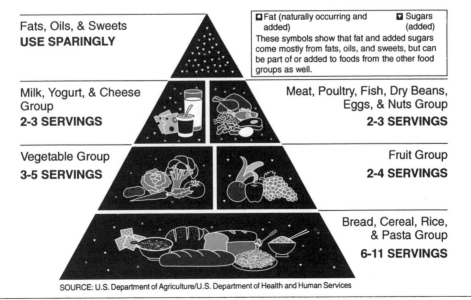

SOURCE: U.S. Department of Agriculture/U.S. Department of Health and Human Services

Figure 2.4 The food guide pyramid.

EATING FOR PERFORMANCE

To help prevent upset stomachs during competition, athletes should

- eat at least 3 to 4 hours before competition;
- avoid foods that are high in fat such as french fries, potato chips, and peanut butter;
- avoid foods that are high in bulk such as lettuce, beans, cabbage, spinach, and nuts;
- avoid foods that are high in sugar such as candy bars, cakes, doughnuts, and honey;
- eat plenty of high-carbohydrate foods that are easily digested, such as pasta, breads, low-fiber cereals, fruit juices, potatoes, and bananas; and
- eat foods that are familiar to the athlete— the pregame meal is no time to try new foods.

adequate time for digestion before a competition.

An adequate diet for an athlete is similar to gasoline for an automobile. It's fuel for performance. To better inform your athletes about the "octane" in their diets, and to learn more about sport drinks and other nutritional issues, read ASEP's *Coaches Guide to Sport Nutrition* (Eisenman, Johnson, and Benson, 1990) for further information.

Ban On Horseplay

Although joking and kidding are basically harmless, horseplay can definitely lead to injury. Establish the rule of "no horseplay" at the start of the season and enforce it at all times. Your team will get more accomplished during practices, and it is less likely that your players will be injured.

Developing an Emergency Plan

The final step in preparing for sports injuries is to develop an emergency plan. To conduct a thorough evaluation of an injured athlete, activate the emergency medical system (EMS), and provide effective first aid, use the following response plan adapted from the American Red Cross:

- Check—*How do I evaluate (**check**) an injured athlete?*
- Call—*How do I activate (**call**) the EMS?*
- Care—*How will first aid **care** be provided?*

How Do I Evaluate *(Check)* an Injured Athlete?

First, your plan needs to specify how you will evaluate an injured athlete. Evaluating injuries is the topic of chapter 4.

How Do I Activate *(Call)* the EMS?

Next, your plan should indicate how to activate the EMS. This section presents a plan for making sure this step is handled efficiently and without confusion. If medical personnel are not present, you should provide first aid care. But, how do you send for medical assistance while you are tending to the athlete? To help everything go more smoothly in the event of an injury, develop a plan for activating the emergency medical system before the season. Here's an effective step-by-step approach you might try.

1. *Delegate the responsibility of seeking medical help* to someone else. This can be either an assistant coach, a parent, or an athlete. But it must be an **adult who is calm and responsible.** Make sure that this person is on hand before every practice and game.
2. *Write out a list of emergency telephone numbers.* This list should be taken to every practice and game and should include phone numbers for the following:

Emergency Numbers

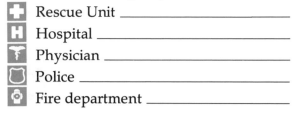

Rescue Unit _____

Hospital _____

Physician _____

Police _____

Fire department _____

If you are traveling to an away game, talk to the host coaches prior to the game about emergency services.

INFORMATION FOR EMERGENCY CALL
(Be prepared to give this information to the EMS dispatcher.)

1. Location
   Street address _____

   City or town _____

   Directions (cross streets, landmarks, etc.) _____

   _____

2. Telephone number from which the call is being made _____

3. Caller's name _____

4. What happened _____

5. How many persons injured _____

6. Condition of victim(s) _____

7. Help (first aid) being given _____

Note: Do not hang up first. Let the EMS dispatcher hang up first.

Figure 2.5 Emergency response card.

INJURY REPORT

Name of athlete _____

Date _____

Time _____

First aider (name) _____

Mechanism of injury _____

_____

_____

Type of injury _____

Anatomical area involved _____

Extent of injury _____

First aid administered _____

_____

_____

Other treatment administered _____

_____

Referral action _____

_____
First aider (Signature)

Figure 2.6 Injury report form.

3. *Take each athlete's emergency information card to every practice and game.* This is especially important if an athlete is unconscious and unable to tell you who you should contact or to give that person's phone number.

4. *Give an emergency response card (see Figure 2.5) to the contact person* calling for emergency assistance. This card will not only help the caller remember to provide critical information to the emergency care staff, but it'll also help the caller keep calm, knowing that everything she or he needs to communicate is spelled out on the card.

5. *Complete an injury report form and keep it on file for any injury* that occurs. It should provide the information requested in the sample shown in Figure 2.6.

How Will First Aid *Care* Be Provided?

Finally, your plan needs to indicate how first aid care will be provided. If medical personnel are on hand at the time of the injury, you should provide assistance to them if needed while they assume the care of the injured athlete. If medical personnel are not present, you should provide first aid care to the extent of your qualifications. Chapters 5 and 6 cover first aid basics and the proper way to move an injured athlete. Part III discusses care of specific injuries.

Handling Minor Injuries

Many injuries don't require emergency medical attention. An athlete who slightly twists an ankle, gets the "wind knocked out" of him or her, or suffers a minor bruise is not in serious condition. However, don't take these noncritical types of injuries lightly. They can severely impair performance and should be

---

EMERGENCY STEPS

If an injury does occur, your emergency plan should follow this sequence:

1. **Check** the athlete's level of consciousness.
2. Send a contact person to activate (**call**) the emergency medical system and **call** the athlete's parents.
3. Send someone to wait for the rescue team and direct them to the injured athlete.
4. Assess (**check**) the injury.
5. Administer first aid (**care**).
6. Assist emergency medical personnel in preparing the athlete for transportation to a medical facility.
7. Appoint someone to go with the athlete if the parents are not available. This person should be responsible, calm, and familiar with the athlete. Assistant coaches or parents are best for this job.
8. Complete an injury report form while the incident is still fresh in your mind.

---

checked closely to ensure that no further complications exist.

For these so-called "minor" injuries, take these steps:

1. Evaluate the injury.
2. Administer first aid.
3. Remove the athlete from participation if the athlete is in a great deal of pain or suffers from a loss of function (can't walk, run, jump, throw, etc.).
4. Contact the athlete's parents.
5. Complete an injury report form while the incident is still fresh in your mind.
6. Discuss the injury with the parents.
7. Suggest that the athlete see a physician to rule out a serious injury.

Sport First Aid Recap

1. The key to controlling and preventing injuries is proper preparation. You'll be better able to control and prevent an injury situation if you prepare yourself to handle it.

2. Studying sports medicine literature, completing first aid and CPR certifications, and attending sports medicine seminars are excellent ways to prepare yourself for handling injuries.

3. Preparing for injuries also requires taking care of administrative paperwork such as parental consent forms and health history forms.

4. As a coach, you should oversee the condition of playing areas and playing equipment. Find and repair any defects before the start of the season.

5. Preparing players for competition can greatly reduce the risk of injury. Athletes should undergo extensive physical examinations and preseason screening to pinpoint any potential health or fitness problems.

6. Preseason conditioning along with warm-up and cool-down exercises are essential for preventing injury.

7. To minimize confusion and ensure that an injured athlete receives prompt medical attention, develop an emergency plan. Outline who is responsible for what duties, how a duty should be carried out, when certain actions should be taken, and what paperwork needs to be completed.

8. You need to teach athletes correct sport skill techniques and repeatedly warn them against techniques that are potentially dangerous.

9. Enforce policies that require athletes to wear protective equipment and refrain from horseplay.

PART II

Basic Sport First Aid Skills

Let's assume that you've enacted all of the planning and preparation measures described in Part I. Now the season has started, and you're watching your team's first scrimmage. You turn and see a player crash to the ground, then you hear the scream of pain. No sports medicine specialist is on hand, and immediate attention is required. What do you do?

a. Run for the hills.
b. Ignore the athlete and continue with practice.
c. Take a deep breath and tend to the athlete.

Surely you answered *c*, but was that actually your first response? If your gut reaction was *a* or *b*, don't worry, you're not alone. Most people would rather walk across hot coals than try to evaluate and treat an injury. They're afraid they'll overlook an injury, make a wrong decision, or give the wrong care.

Preparation is the key to eliminating the anxiety over administering sport first aid. Just like your athletes, you'll be more confident and successful if you master the basic skills and learn the basic rules and strategies. Chapter 3 will help you develop a basic knowledge of anatomy, which is essential to your being able to administer appropriate sport first aid. Also, the Glossary in the back of the book (pages 171-174) will help you learn the terms commonly used in sports medicine. Once you've developed a sound knowledge base, you'll better understand the guidelines for evaluating injuries presented in chapter 4.

Just as you would develop strategies to break a team's player-to-player defense, the sport first aid tactics outlined in chapter 5 will help you handle any common sport first aid problem. These are the basic formations, if you will, from which you will run all of your specific emergency plays.

Finally, in chapter 6, you'll learn ways to assist in safely moving an injured athlete. The secrets here are caution and proper technique, depending on the type of injury incurred.

The chapters in this section will help you take the guesswork and fear out of administering sport first aid. With these common guidelines understood, you'll find evaluating and treating injured athletes easier and less intimidating.

CHAPTER 3

Anatomy and Sport Injury Terminology

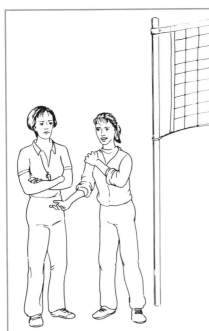

Imagine that you are coaching a varsity volleyball team. A player returns from seeing the physician and tells you, "The doctor said I have a recurrent subluxating shoulder and he'd like me to do some rotator cuff strengthening." You hope that the athlete will explain further, so you don't have to suffer the embarrassment of her realizing that you haven't a clue as to what she's talking about.

Recurrent subluxation? Rotator cuff? If you're unfamiliar with basic anatomical terminology, these words probably sound foreign to you.

In this chapter you'll explore anatomical and sport injury terminology. With a better understanding of these areas, you'll be able to

1. improve your understanding of physicians' diagnoses and orders, and
2. better relate an athlete's symptoms and problems to parents, guardians, or sports medicine professionals.

Before we get into evaluating and treating specific sport injuries, let's review basic human anatomy. As you know, the body can be divided into several systems, and within these systems are several body constituents. Each system is vital to supporting life. Each is also prone to certain injuries and illnesses.

Musculoskeletal System

Let's look first at the foundation of the body—the musculoskeletal system. As the name indicates, this system is made up of bones, muscles, and joints.

Bones

The skeleton (bones) is the body's infrastructure. Its two primary functions are

- to support the body, and
- to protect important organs such as the brain, lungs, and heart.

As illustrated in Figure 3.1, the bones are effectively positioned and sized to serve these two functions.

Muscles

Muscles are fibrous elastic tissues that move bones. The most common muscle groups injured in sport are as follows (see Figure 3.2):

Rotator cuff—located on the shoulder blade, these muscles are involved in throwing motions.

Quadriceps—located on the front of the thigh, these muscles straighten the knee and move or bend the thigh forward.

Hamstring—located on the back of the thigh, these muscles bend the knee and move the thigh backward.

Calf—located on the back of the lower leg, these muscles point the foot down and also help bend the knee.

Ligaments

Ligaments are bands of tissue that typically serve to connect bones at joints. Their major duty is to hold the bones together; they are therefore extremely important to joint stability.

Tendons

Tendons are fibrous elastic tissues that attach muscle to bone.

These tendons are commonly injured in sport (see Figure 3.3):

Achilles (heel)

Patellar (kneecap)

Biceps (upper arm)

Rotator cuff (shoulder)

Cartilage

Cartilage is a gristly type of tissue most often found on the ends of bones. It helps absorb the shock of bones hitting each other and reduces the friction of bones rubbing together.

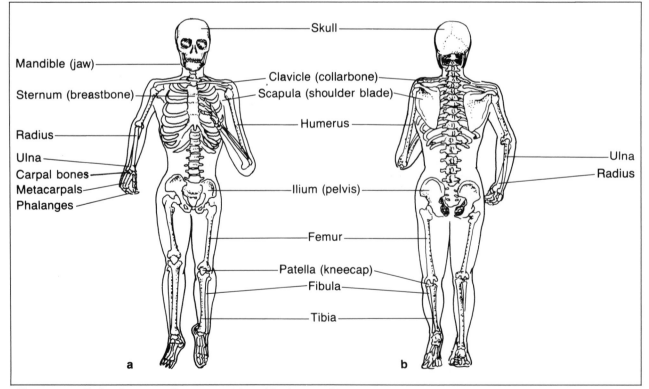

Figure 3.1 Skeletal system. Front view (a) and back view (b).

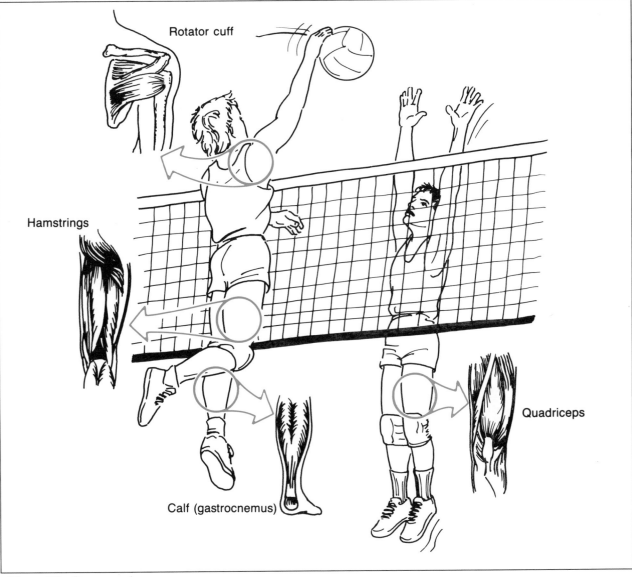

Figure 3.2 Four muscle groups.

Bursa

Bursa are small, fluid-filled sacs located between bones, muscles, tendons, and other tissues. They help to reduce friction between tissues.

Joints

The body, however, would be immobile if not for the movement afforded by the joints—the places where bones join. Joints in the body are made up of ligaments, tendons, cartilage, and bursa (see Figure 3.4). Primary joints include the knee, elbow, shoulder, and ankle.

Neurological System

As a coach, you appreciate the importance of the mental aspect of your sport. Furthermore, you know how nerves can affect your players' performance. So the neurological system—the body's control center—is a key component of the body that you must understand (see Figure 3.5).

The brain is the control center that coordinates the functioning of all body tissues. Digestion, breathing and heart rates, muscle contraction, and most other bodily functions depend on signals from the brain. The brain sends these directions to the tissues through a system of nerves.

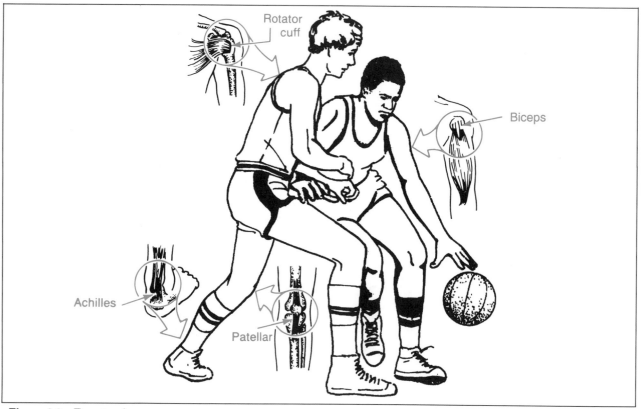

Figure 3.3   Four tendons.

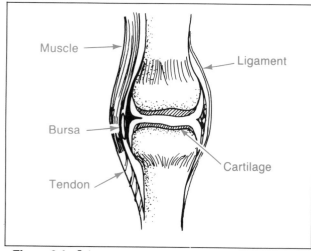

Figure 3.4   Joint structure.

The spinal cord is the main trunk from which the nerves branch. It is protected by a column of bones called the spinal column. The bones, or vertebrae, of the spinal column are held together by ligaments (see Figure 3.6). Through the nerves the brain can send out electrical impulses to the various tissues to make them function. The brain also receives feedback from the tissues through the nerves.

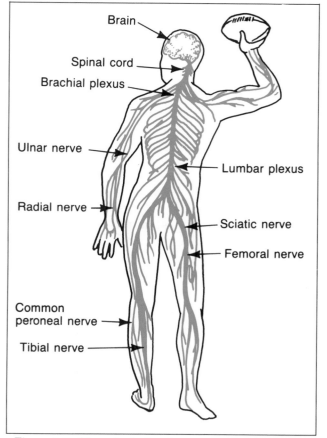

Figure 3.5   Neurological system.

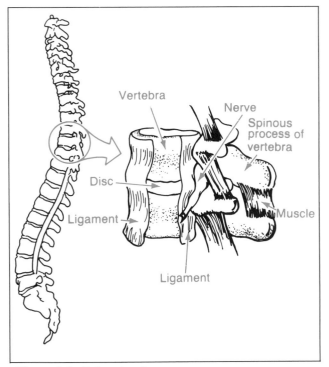

Figure 3.6 Spine structures.

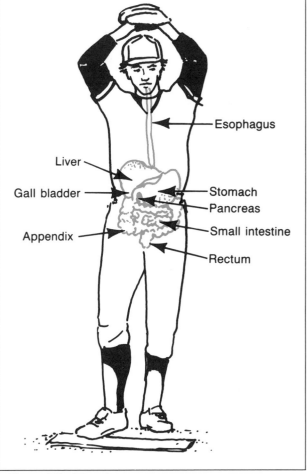

Figure 3.7 Digestive system.

Digestive System

The digestive system is the body's energy supply center. The organs that compose it assist in breaking down food into energy substances that the muscles and other tissues can then use (see Figure 3.7). This system is very sensitive to the anxiety athletes experience before engaging in sports events. So the terms "butterflies in the stomach" or "choking under pressure" may describe an athlete's actual physical sensations!

Circulatory and Respiratory Systems

With the digestive system as the energy supplier, the circulatory and respiratory systems combine to serve as the body's energy releaser. These two systems work together to supply the oxygen the body needs to sustain life. Oxygen helps release the energy from food to fuel-using tissues. Shut off the oxygen supply to the body, and the body shuts down.

The circulatory system consists of the blood-transporting network shown in Figure 3.8. Note how the central pump in this network, the heart, must provide blood to every part of the body.

The respiratory system is the body's air-transporting network. The respiratory organs are located in the head and chest area (see Figure 3.9). Though less extensive than the circulatory system, that doesn't mean that the respiratory system is less important. All you have to do is hold your breath and pinch your nose shut for a while to realize how much we rely on our ability to breathe.

The Respiratory and Circulatory Systems at Work

A person breathes in oxygen-filled air through the nose, mouth, or both. This air then travels down the windpipe or trachea until it reaches the lungs. Inside the lungs, the oxygen passes through tiny sacs called aveoli and into thin

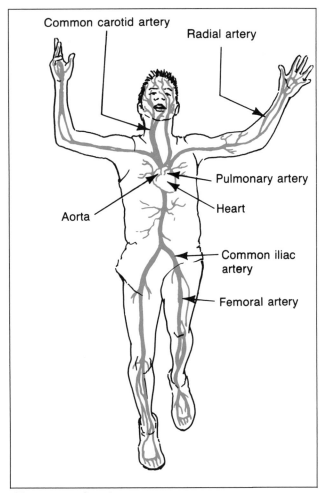

Figure 3.8 Circulatory system.

dioxide. The capillaries pick up the carbon dioxide, and this blood, called venous or low-oxygen blood, returns to the heart via the veins. The heart pumps the low-oxygen blood to the lungs, where it gets rid of the carbon dioxide and picks up new supplies of oxygen from the air.

A synopsis of this circulatory cycle is illustrated in Figure 3.10.

Urinary System

After the energy is supplied (by digestion) and released for the body to use (by circulation and respiration), the by-products need to be disposed of. The urinary system rids the body of waste products from energy breakdown. The organs shown in Figure 3.11 participate in this process.

Waste products are brought to the kidneys through the blood (circulatory system). The kidneys filter out the waste products from the blood and combine them with water to make urine. The urine is released from the kidneys and travels through the ureters to the bladder. The bladder stores the urine until it is released from the body.

blood vessels called capillaries. The capillaries join together into large blood vessels called pulmonary veins, which take the oxygen-filled blood to the heart.

The heart pumps the oxygen-filled blood through the arteries to the body tissues. In the tissues, oxygen is used to release energy and is broken down to a waste product called carbon

Interdependence of the Body Systems

As you can see, the body's systems and organs depend on each other. The way one system functions will affect every other system. That is why an injury or illness in any body part can cause problems with other parts.

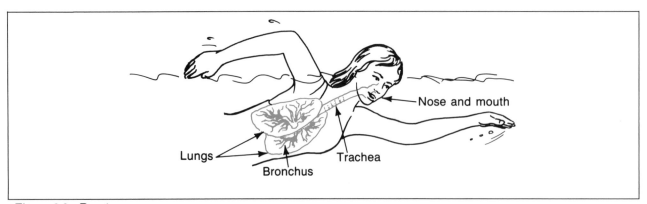

Figure 3.9 Respiratory system.

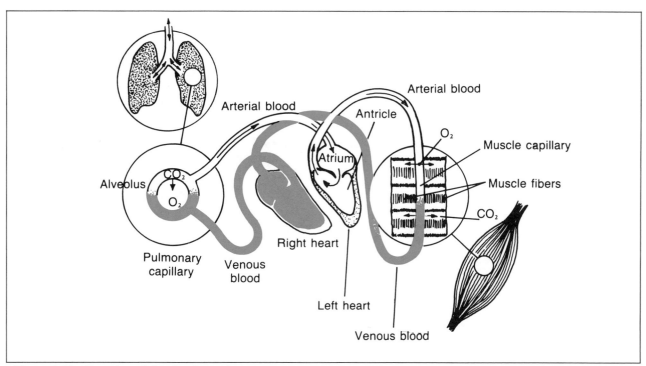

Figure 3.10 Function of the circulorespiratory system.

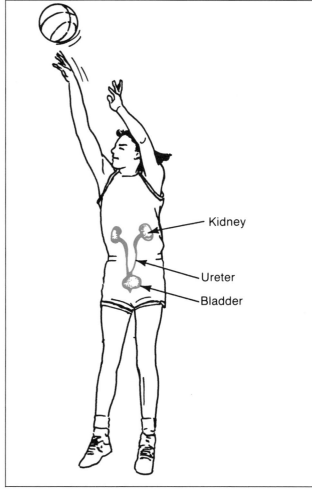

Figure 3.11 Urinary system.

With a greater appreciation of the body's makeup, let's look at some of the injuries that can alter the body's functioning. Specifically, we'll examine those injuries most likely to occur in sports.

Sport Injury

Athletes can be stricken with any number of physical ailments. So we need a classification system to communicate effectively about sport injury. And this classification system is essential for prevention, identification, and treatment of each particular problem.

All injuries and illnesses can be categorized according to the length of time they take to develop. These are the two most common time-related classes of injuries:

Acute—occurring suddenly
Examples: Broken bones, cuts, bruises, appendicitis, etc.

Chronic—developing or lasting over a long period
Examples: Shinsplints, tennis elbow, diabetes, epilepsy, etc.

But knowing only the term of onset is hardly sufficient information. After all, first aid for an acute bone fracture differs markedly from that for an acute incision. So, to further clarify the various types of injuries, we'll classify them according to the type of body structures that are damaged. These are the two most common categories for body constituents:

Soft tissues—nerves, blood vessels, muscles, skin, organs, tendons, cartilage, ligaments, bursa, etc.
Examples: Pulled muscles, bruises, etc.

Hard tissues—bones
Examples: Fractures, stress fractures, etc.

Injuries can also be classified according to how they occur. This information is extremely helpful when checking for injury. It can provide clues as to the type of injury. Sport injuries are often caused by the following mechanisms:

Direct blow—A direct blow to a specific body part can cause bleeding, superficial and deep tissue bruising, broken bones, or joint injuries.

Colliding with another athlete or with sports equipment and falling on a hard surface are common examples of a direct blow mechanism in sport (see Figure 3.12).

Torsion—A torsion injury is a twisting injury. Examples of this mechanism include cutting and pivoting motions in football and basketball and twisting of arms or legs in wrestling. Torsion or twisting often results in joint injuries or broken bones (see Figure 3.13).

Shearing—A shearing injury is a friction injury caused by two surfaces rubbing together. Contact between the skin and the ground can cause a shearing injury during a softball or baseball slide. Shearing usually causes skin injuries, but can affect other tissues as well (see Figure 3.14).

Using our time-related and body-structure classifications, we can then examine the similarities between injuries that fall into one of these four categories: acute soft-tissue, chronic soft-tissue, acute hard-tissue, and chronic

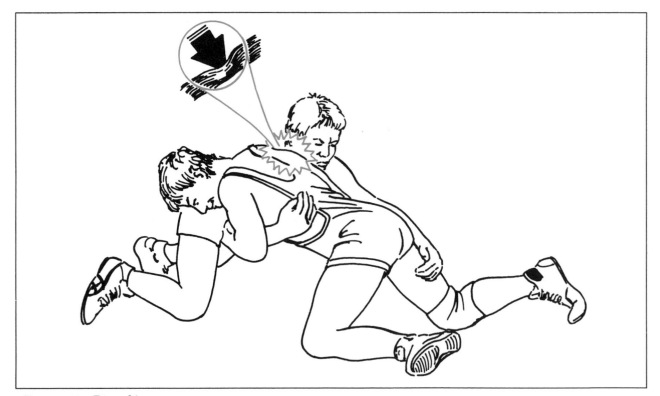

Figure 3.12   Direct blow.

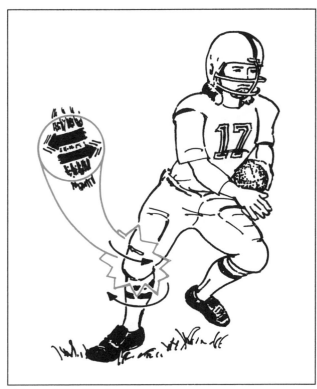

Figure 3.13 Torsion.

hard-tissue. So let's take a look at specific injuries that fit these descriptions.

Acute Soft-Tissue Injuries

Many sport injuries occur suddenly to soft tissues like skin, muscle, ligaments, tendons, organs, blood vessels, and nerves. There are several different types of acute soft-tissue injuries:

- Contusions
- Abrasions
- Punctures
- Cuts
  - Lacerations
  - Incisions
  - Avulsions
- Sprains
- Strains
- Cartilage tears
- Dislocations and subluxations

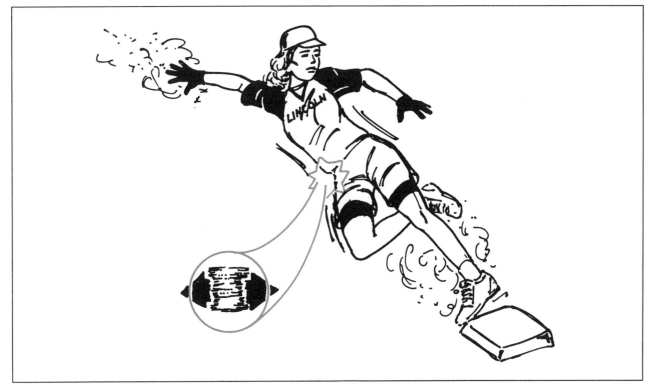

Figure 3.14 Shearing or tearing.

Contusions

Contusions, or bruises, are a common soft-tissue injury. As a result of a direct blow, tissue and capillaries are damaged and lose fluid and blood. This causes pain, swelling, and discoloration. Contusions to the skin are minor, but contusions to bone and muscle can cause loss of function (see Figure 3.15). Contusions to the heart, lungs, brain, kidneys, or other organs can be life-threatening.

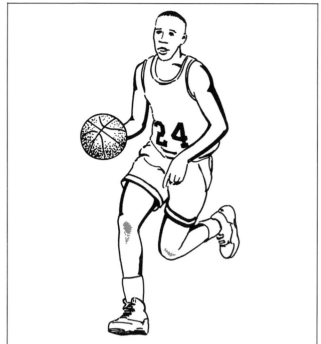

Figure 3.16   Leg abrasion.

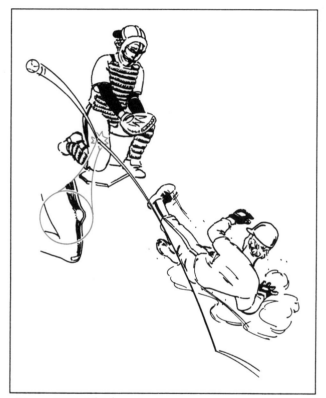

Figure 3.15   Thigh contusion.

Abrasions

In abrasions, friction or scraping injures the outer layer of a tissue. Most abrasions occur to the skin, such as turf burns and strawberries (see Figure 3.16). The cornea, or outer layer of the eye, can also be abraded or scratched by dust and other objects.

Punctures

Punctures are narrow stab wounds to the skin and internal organs. You've probably seen skin punctures caused by track spikes, wood splin-

ters, fishing hooks, or nails, as shown in Figure 3.17. Although superficial skin punctures may not bleed much, they should not be treated lightly because bacteria and other materials may collect in the wound and cause infection.

Lungs and other internal organs can be punctured by sharp objects such as javelins. These injuries are life threatening and require prompt treatment.

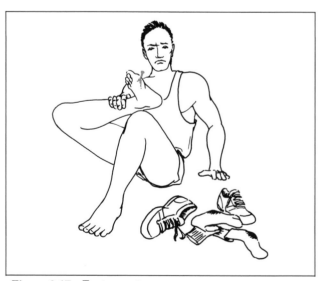

Figure 3.17   Foot puncture.

Cuts

Soft tissue may be cut or torn in three general ways. Following are brief descriptions and illustrations of these types of cuts: lacerations, incisions, and avulsions.

Lacerations. Lacerations are jagged soft-tissue cuts (see Figure 3.18) caused by a blow from a blunt object. They are deeper than abrasions and cause steady bleeding. For example, a basketball player can suffer a laceration above the eye after catching an elbow to the face.

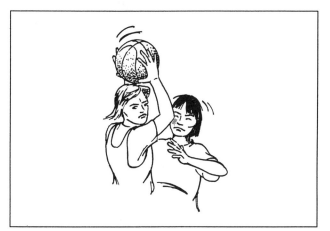

Figure 3.18 Facial laceration.

Incisions. Incisions are smooth cuts caused by very sharp glass or metal objects (see Figure 3.19). They usually bleed heavily and quickly. Coaches can help athletes avoid most situations where incisions occur by conducting regular thorough inspections of facilities and equipment.

Avulsions. Avulsions are complete tissue tears. Athletes who wear earrings are especially prone to avulsions of the earlobe (see Figure 3.20). Also, athletes wearing rings can suffer finger avulsions. That's why wearing jewelry should be forbidden in every type of athletic event.

Sprains

Sprains occur when ligaments are stretched, torn, or both (see Figure 3.21). They are caused by a direct blow or twisting/torsion.

A ligament sprain can cause a joint to lose its stability. Remember, ligaments support a

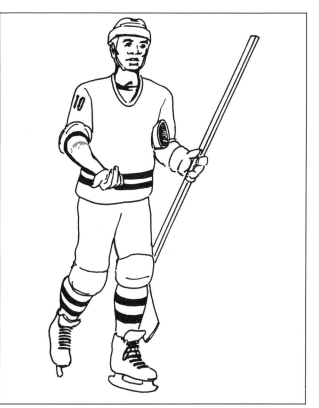

Figure 3.19 Arm incision.

joint by holding the bones together. Without support, the bones will not stay in place. Once stretched or torn, ligaments do not necessarily regain their original length and may heal lengthened or stretched. That is why sprained ankles and knees can be reinjured.

Strains

If a muscle or tendon is forcefully shortened or stretched, it can become strained. A strain,

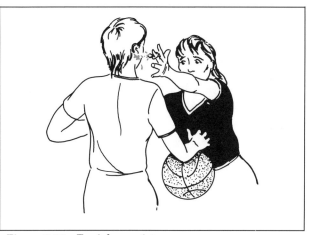

Figure 3.20 Ear lobe avulsion.

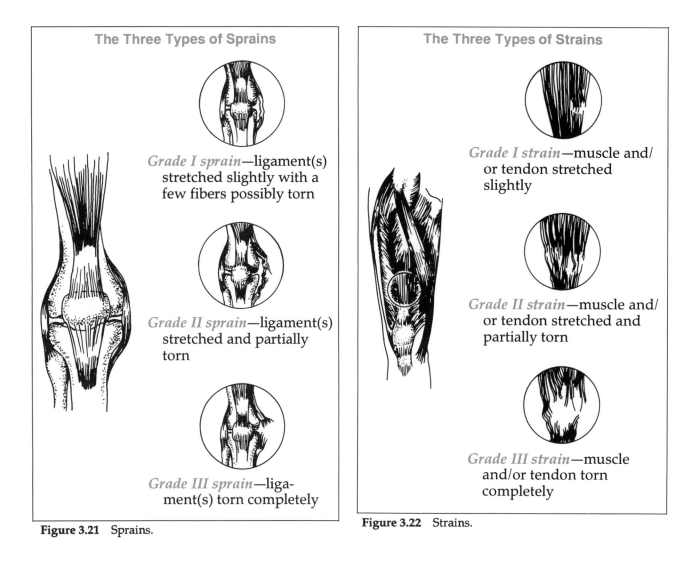

The Three Types of Sprains

Grade I sprain—ligament(s) stretched slightly with a few fibers possibly torn

Grade II sprain—ligament(s) stretched and partially torn

Grade III sprain—ligament(s) torn completely

Figure 3.21   Sprains.

The Three Types of Strains

Grade I strain—muscle and/ or tendon stretched slightly

Grade II strain—muscle and/ or tendon stretched and partially torn

Grade III strain—muscle and/or tendon torn completely

Figure 3.22   Strains.

like a sprain, is a stretching or tearing injury (see Figure 3.22); strains, however, occur only in muscles and tendons (you'll recall that sprains occur only in ligaments). If severe, a strain can disrupt a muscle's and/or tendon's ability to move the bones.

Cartilage Tears

As you'll remember, cartilage covers the ends of bones and reduces shock and friction. If the bones of a joint are twisted and compressed, they may pinch and tear the cartilage. This injury frequently occurs in the knee (see Figure 3.23).

Dislocations and Subluxations

Sometimes when a joint is hit or twisted, the bones move out of position. We say the bones

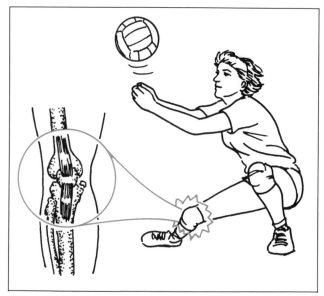

Figure 3.23   Knee cartilage tear.

of a joint are dislocated if they stay out of place until a physician repositions them. If the bones "pop out" of place but immediately "pop" back in, a subluxation has occurred. The most common dislocations and subluxations in sports occur to the shoulder (see Figure 3.24), elbow, fingers, and kneecap.

Dislocations and subluxations most often injure the soft tissues around a joint. For example, ligaments are often sprained during dislocations and subluxations because their tissues are stretched or torn when the bones move out of place. Bones can also break during these injuries, although this is not a common occurrence. That is why dislocations and subluxations are classified as acute soft-tissue injuries.

Chronic Soft-Tissue Injuries

Chronic injuries to the muscles, tendons, and bursa are caused by repeated blows, overstretching, repeated friction, or overuse. These injuries typically occur in athletes who are weak and inflexible or who exercise excessively.

Chronic Muscle Strain

If a muscle is repeatedly overworked or overstretched, a chronic strain can result. This type

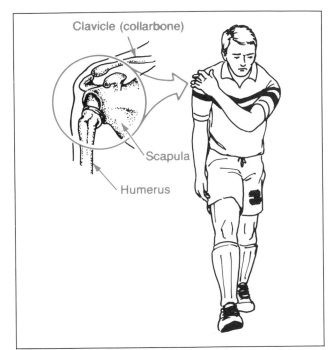

Figure 3.24 Shoulder dislocation.

of injury develops over a period of weeks or months and can last just as long. Such strains are different from acute strains, because they are not caused by one specific episode of injury, such as pulling up from a sprint.

Bursitis

Bursa can become swollen and sore if they suffer from repeated blows or irritation. Elbow and kneecap (see Figure 3.25) bursitis are the most common types in sports.

Tendinitis

Just as bursa become irritated, tendons can also be irritated by repeated overstretching or overuse. This most often occurs in tendons that are tight or weak. The patella (kneecap), Achilles (heel), biceps, and rotator cuff (shoulder) tendons are especially prone to irritation in sports. Inflexible and weak patellar and Achilles tendons can be overstressed by repeated running and jumping activities. The biceps and rotator cuff tendons are usually overstressed when an athlete throws with a weak and inflexible shoulder.

Acute Hard-Tissue (Bone) Injuries

We've all seen a player get hit or land hard on the ground, and have perhaps even heard the snap of a bone. Although the skeleton is strong, there is a limit to how much punishment it can take. Let's now look at those types of injuries to bone that often occur before an athlete realizes what's happened.

Fractures

Sticks and stones aren't the only things that can break bones. An aggressive tackle or a poorly executed slide can do it also. In sport, bones that are twisted or hit too hard can break or fracture. You should be able to recognize the various types of fractures (see Figure 3.26).

Closed Fractures. Closed fractures are by far the most common fractures that occur in sport. Although they are most often detected because they cause a noticeable deformity, not all fractures cause deformity. Two common closed fractures in sport are as follows:

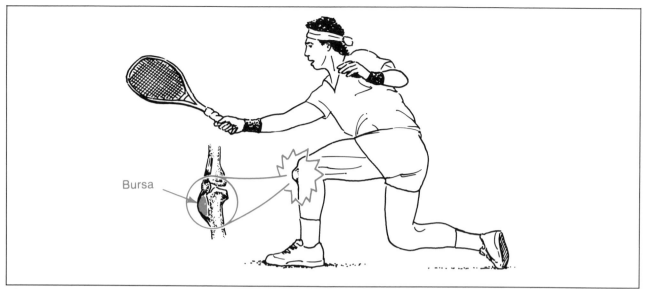

Figure 3.25   Knee bursitis.

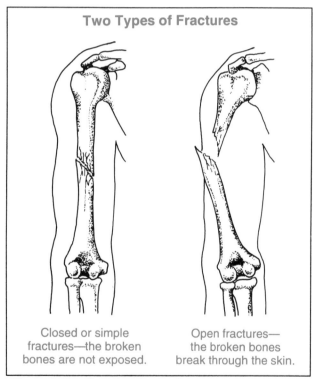

Figure 3.26   Closed and open fractures.

Avulsion fractures—these occur when sprained ligaments pull off a piece of bone. This can frequently take place in the ankle (see figure 3.27) and finger.

Epiphyseal (growth plate) fractures—growth plates at the ends of bones are soft and especially prone to injury. A fracture of the epiphysis can affect a bone's growth. A common growth plate fracture occurs in the elbow of baseball pitchers, as shown in Figure 3.28.

Open Fractures.   A rare occurrence in sport, an open fracture is easily detected by a deformity and open wound. You will be able to see at least one of the bones poking through the skin. Because the bone and muscle tissues are exposed, the first aid provider must take great care to cover open fractures with sterile gauze.

Chronic Hard-Tissue (Bone) Injuries

Subjected to repeated wear and tear over an extended period of time, bones can suffer chronic conditions that can lead to cracking and abnormal boney formations. Perhaps the most common types of chronic bone injury are stress fractures and arthritis. Arthritis is fairly uncommon in high school athletes, but stress fractures do occur, especially in basketball and track athletes.

Stress Fractures

If a bone suffers repeated stress or shock, it can eventually crack. This is called a stress fracture. Athletes especially prone to stress fractures include runners who run more than 5 miles every day without taking a day of rest

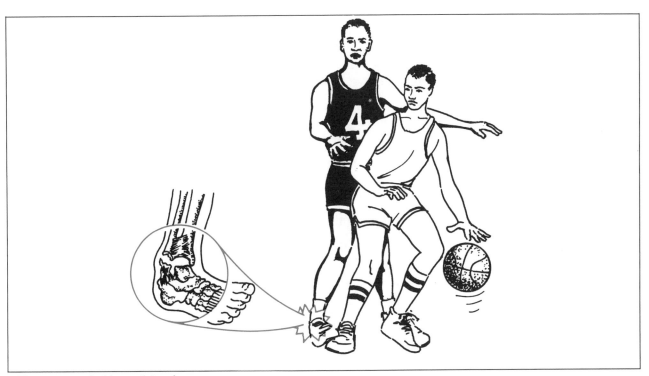

Figure 3.27   Ankle avulsion fracture.

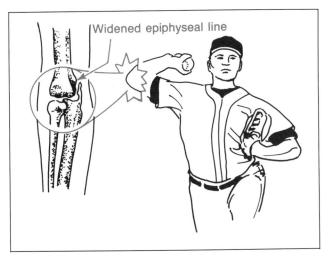

Widened epiphyseal line

Figure 3.28   Elbow epiphyseal/growth plate fracture.

and baseball pitchers who throw at full speed on a daily basis.

These are just a few of the many injuries that you may encounter as a coach. For more information on specific injuries, see the chapters in Part III that apply to the particular conditions that concern you.

Sport First Aid Recap

1. The body consists of many systems that depend on each other to function effectively.

2. The neurological, digestive, circulatory, and respiratory systems all support the musculoskeletal system, the main system utilized in sport.

3. Injuries can roughly be categorized by the length of time it takes for them to occur (acute vs. chronic) and the structures involved (soft-tissue vs. hard-tissue).

4. Contusions are bruising injuries to either soft or hard tissue.

5. Lacerations, abrasions, and punctures generally affect the skin, but also occur in the eye and internal organs.

6. Ligaments connect bone to bone and help hold them together.

7. Sprains or stretching and tearing injuries of ligaments are common in sport, especially at the ankle, fingers, and knee.

8. Tendons attach muscle to bone.

9. Strains (stretching and tearing injuries of muscle and tendons) are also common in sport and can be either acute (sudden) or chronic.

10. Closed fractures are the most common hard-tissue injuries in sport.

11. In subluxations, bones in a joint temporarily move out of place, whereas in dislocations the bones stay out of place. In both types of injury, the ligaments are also injured.

CHAPTER 4

Injury Evaluation

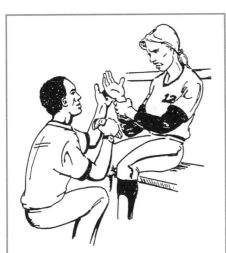

Jackie Hayes slides into home, tying the score of the first-round state tournament softball game. When she reaches the dugout, though, she is clutching her right hand and jumping up and down. Coach Jones grabs Jackie's hand and immediately yanks off her batting glove. He can't really detect anything wrong with the hand, but Jackie complains that her thumb hurts. Because he can't actually see an injury and doesn't know what else to do, he tightly tapes Jackie's thumb and puts her back into the game to catch. After catching one pitch, Jackie collapses with pain.

If you don't have any procedures established for conducting an injury evaluation, you might overlook an injury. And if you have nothing in your first aid guidelines about moving an injured athlete or allowing a hurt player to resume participation, you may cause further harm to the athlete.

This chapter won't tell you how to diagnose an injury, but it may help you prevent an injury from getting worse. And it will certainly help you more effectively address the next injury situation that you encounter.

Preevaluation Steps

As you run out onto the court, field, or track to attend to an injured athlete, you must have your thoughts in order. Before you evaluate the injury, your primary concern is to **check** the athlete's

1. safety,
2. position, and
3. equipment.

Safety

When an athlete goes down, your immediate response should be to protect him or her from further harm. First, instruct all other players and bystanders to leave the athlete alone. They can cause further injury by trying to move an athlete. You may even need to reroute traffic or spectators to make sure everyone stays clear of the athlete.

Try to calm the athlete and keep him or her from moving until you have evaluated the injury. Most injured athletes roll around or jump up and down because of pain; this extra movement may cause further harm.

Position

Always let the medical personnel move a seriously injured athlete. However, if you must do it, make sure you know the guidelines and procedures outlined in chapter 6 of this book.

For a Seriously Injured Athlete

DO NOT . . .

. . . move the athlete unless he or she is at risk of further injury.

. . . alter the athlete's position unless it prevents you from evaluating or treating the injury.

Equipment

Refer back to the opening of this chapter. In the case of Jackie Hayes and her thumb injury, should Coach Jones have removed her batting glove? Many coaches face a similar question when trying to decide whether to remove the shoe of an athlete with an ankle injury. What should you do in this situation?

On Removing Equipment

DO NOT . . .

. . . remove equipment if doing so will further harm an athlete. You'll waste valuable time that you should use to **check** and **care** for the injury. The only exception is a football helmet face mask. If a face mask is preventing you from checking an athlete's airway or breathing, simply cut (a scalpel or sharp knife works best) the straps or tabs on the side of the helmet that are holding the mask in place. Then you can carefully pull back the mask to the position shown in Figure 4.1. Do not use bolt cutters on the tabs because they will jar the athlete's head. Another alternative is to use a face shield (Figure 4.6) that includes a breathing tube. In this case, slip the shield under the face mask, make sure the breathing tube sticks up through the face mask, and begin rescue breathing or CPR. This will ultimately save time and cause less jostling of the athlete.

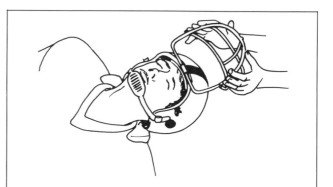

Figure 4.1   Face mask removal.

Evaluating (*Checking*) the Athlete

Having considered the athlete's safety, position, and equipment, you can conduct your evaluation. As you move quickly toward the injured athlete to evaluate the injury, follow these steps:

1. *Remain calm.* An athlete who is in pain will be upset. You will only upset the athlete more by getting excited, making your evaluation more difficult.
2. *Remember any preexisting health problems.* Does the athlete have a history of asthma, heart problems, kidney disorders, neurological problems, diabetes, or seizures? Has he or she ever suffered a similar injury? This information provides clues to what may be wrong with the athlete. It will also dictate the care you provide.
3. *Recall the mechanism of injury,* or how the injury occurred. Was there a direct hit to a certain area of the body? Was a joint or body part twisted? This information gives you insight into what type of injury you're dealing with.

Once you reach the athlete, **check** whether he or she is conscious or unconscious. Do this by first calling out the athlete's name; if you get no response, then pinch the skin between the athlete's thumb and index finger and see whether he or she responds. If the athlete still does not respond, send someone to **call** for emergency medical assistance.

Primary Survey

After determining an athlete's level of consciousness and sending for emergency medical assistance, perform a primary survey to **check** his or her vital signs (breathing and heart rates). Think of it as checking the ABCs:

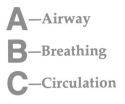

A—Airway

B—Breathing

C—Circulation

ABCs for the Conscious Athlete

If the athlete is conscious, don't assume that he or she has an adequate airway, normal breathing, or a normal pulse (heart rate). **Check** each of the ABCs to be sure.

Airway

Check the airway by listening for any gasping or choking noises, by checking for the universal choking signal (the athlete grabs his or her throat), and also by asking the athlete, "Can you speak?" If the athlete can talk, you can assume that for the time being, the airway is open.

If the athlete is unable to speak, ask, "Are you choking?" If he or she responds by nodding "yes," or by grasping the throat (the universal choking sign), you must provide first aid **care**, in this case the Heimlich maneuver. This procedure is described on pages 70-72.

Breathing

If the athlete is having difficulty breathing, but is able to speak continue with your injury survey until you determine what is causing the breathing problems. An athlete may have had the "wind knocked out" and be unable to catch his or her breath. This and other breathing conditions are further discussed in chapter 7.

Circulation

At this point, **check** the pulse (heart rate) at either the wrist (radial) or neck (carotid). Although the carotid pulse is easier to feel than the radial, be careful not to push too hard, or else you may reduce the blood supply to the athlete's brain. When taking a pulse, you will try to determine the rate, regularity, and strength of the heartbeat. Because your thumb has its own pulse, be sure to use your other fingers to take someone else's pulse. See Figure 4.2 for correct positioning.

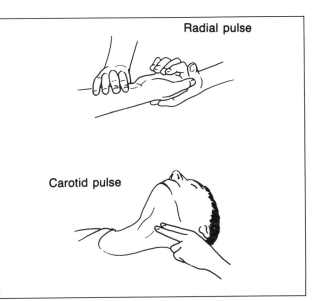

Figure 4.2 Two pulses.

Remember, if the athlete has been active, the pulse and breathing rates will be faster than the resting rates. Table 4.1 provides the normal resting heart and breathing rates for various ages. If the athlete is breathing normally and has a normal pulse, you can proceed to the secondary survey (pp. 48-50).

Table 4.1   Normal Resting Heart and Breathing Rates

Age group	Heart rate*	Breathing rate**
Children (5 to 12 years)	60-120	20
Adolescents (12 to 18 years)	75-85	12-20
Adults	60-100	12-15

*Beats per minute

**Breaths per minute

ABCs for the Unconscious Athlete

Tim Watts is slammed to the mat during a wrestling match. After hitting the mat, Tim's body immediately goes limp. The referee stops the match and Coach Thompson **checks** Tim's responsiveness by calling out his name and tapping him on the shoulder. Tim doesn't respond. Coach Thompson wants to make sure that Tim has an airway and is breathing properly, but Tim is lying facedown on the mat. What should Coach Thompson do?

Airway

The position of an unconscious athlete is a concern when you're trying to **check** the airway. You must be able to either feel the athlete's breath or see breathing movements.

If the athlete is lying on his or her back, lean over and place your ear and cheek next to the athlete's nose and mouth as in Figure 4.3.

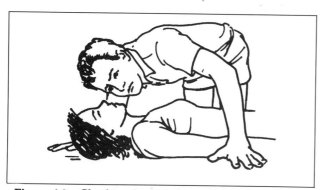

Figure 4.3 Checking for breathing.

While in this position you will attempt to do the following:

1. *Look* for breathing movements. Is the chest rising and falling? Is the breathing shallow or deep?
2. *Listen* for breathing sounds coming from the nose or mouth. Are there any unusual sounds such as gasping, wheezing, or labored breathing?
3. *Feel* with your cheek whether air is moving in and out of the nose or mouth.

If the athlete is lying on his or her side or stomach, you must be more resourceful. Here are three ways that you might check for breathing in such instances.

1. *Place your hand near the athlete's mouth.* Feel for breathing. At the same time, watch the rib cage for respiratory movements.
2. *Place a mirror near the athlete's nose and mouth.* The mirror will fog if the athlete is breathing.
3. *Move the athlete.* If all else fails, move the athlete. Always assume that the athlete has a neck or spinal injury; make sure the athlete's head is stabilized and that the whole body is moved as a unit. In chapter 6 you'll learn the specific guidelines and procedures for moving an unconscious athlete.

Opening an Airway. If you do not see, hear, or feel the athlete breathing, attempt to establish an airway. There are two methods for doing this:

Head Tilt/Chin Lift (if no spinal cord injury is suspected; see Figure 4.4)
1. Place your fingertips just below the athlete's chin and gently lift the chin forward.
2. Stabilize the athlete's head with your other hand on the forehead.
3. Look, listen, and feel for breathing.

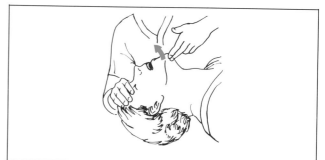

Figure 4.4 Head tilt/chin lift.

Chin Lift (for unconscious athletes with suspected neck or spinal cord injuries caused by a direct blow or torsion injury; see Figure 4.5):
1. Without tilting the head, place your fingertips just below the athlete's chin and gently lift the chin forward.
2. Look, listen, and feel for breathing.
3. If you still don't see, hear, or feel breathing, let the chin relax and then try the chin lift again.
4. If this still doesn't work, try tilting the head very slightly while trying to lift the chin. This may be enough to open the airway.

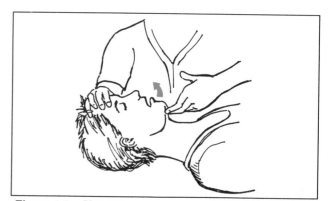

Figure 4.5 Chin lift.

Breathing

Once you've established an airway through either the head tilt/chin lift or the chin lift only method, what do you do if the athlete still isn't breathing? You must attempt to ventilate or inflate the lungs.

Face Shield. Before we discuss how to administer rescue breathing, let's talk about face shields. With the rise in AIDS and hepatitis B, it is recommended that you carry a face shield in your first aid kit. This shield can be placed over an athlete's nose and mouth to act as a barrier between you and the athlete. There are several different types available (see Figure 4.6).

To perform rescue breathing, follow these steps:

1. Place a face shield over the athlete's nose and mouth.

2. Hold the athlete's head with either the head tilt/chin lift or the chin lift only.

3. If the shield does not seal off the nose, pinch the nose shut and lift the chin (using head tilt/chin lift or chin lift only) as shown in Figure 4.7.

4. Seal your mouth over the opening to the athlete's mouth.

5. Give two slow, full breaths for adults or two slow, gentle breaths for children.

6. Watch to see whether the chest rises during the breaths.

7. Next, turn your head to look, listen, and feel for the breath to come out of the athlete's nose and mouth.

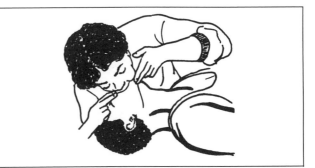

Figure 4.7 Attempting to ventilate the lungs.

8. If the air doesn't go in, reposition the athlete's head (head tilt/chin lift), or in the case of a suspected spine injury, attempt the chin lift method again.

9. If air still doesn't go in, you must start first aid for a blocked airway—the Heimlich maneuver (see pages 70-71).

Circulation

After you've given the two full breaths, check the athlete's pulse to determine whether the heart is beating. This should be done while you look, listen, and feel for the athlete to exhale or breathe out the two full breaths. Check the circulation as follows:

1. Using the hand nearest the athlete's body, place your index and middle fingertips over the athlete's Adam's apple.

2. Slide your fingertips back and up onto the groove along the side of the neck. Use the index and middle finger, but not the thumb, to gently apply pressure over the carotid artery (see Figure 4.2 on page 45).

3. Check the pulse for 5-10 seconds.

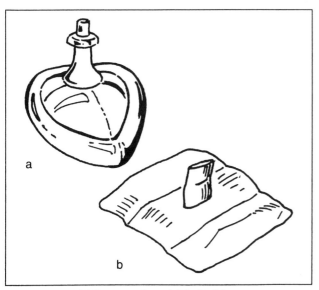

Figure 4.6 (a) Face mask and (b) shield.

WHEN THE ABCs = 0

If there is no breathing or pulse after you've checked the ABCs, you should take the following actions:

1. Make sure someone has activated the emergency medical system.
2. Begin cardiopulmonary resuscitation (CPR).
3. Scan quickly for any profuse bleeding while you perform CPR.
4. If there is bleeding, designate someone to apply sterile gauze and direct pressure over the area while you give CPR.

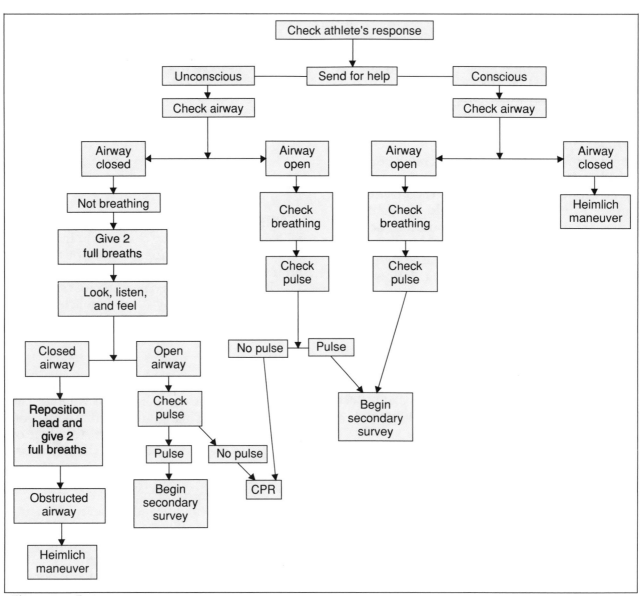

Figure 4.8 Primary survey summary.

Primary Survey Summary

When an athlete goes down with an injury, you should do as follows (see Figure 4.8):

1. **Check** whether the athlete is conscious or unconscious.
2. **Call** for emergency medical assistance.
3. If unconscious, **check** the athlete's ABCs:

   Airway—use head tilt/chin lift or chin lift only.

   Breathing—look, listen, and feel for breathing. If none, give two full breaths.

   Circulation—check carotid (neck) pulse.
4. If the athlete is conscious and able to talk, **check** these functions:

Breathing—for irregularities

Pulse—for heart or circulation problems

5. If both breathing and pulse are normal, begin the secondary survey to locate and **check** the extent of the injury.

Secondary Survey

When an injured athlete is conscious and has normal breathing and heart rates, you should perform a secondary survey (**check**). During this secondary survey, you will pinpoint the nature, site, and severity of an injury. As with the primary survey, you should follow a standard pattern to make the evaluation more thorough. The steps in the secondary survey are easy to remember with the acronym HIT:

H—History

I—Inspection

T—Touch

History

If an athlete is injured, the success of your evaluation will depend on your getting a history of how the injury happened. Your goals in obtaining the history of an injury are to determine its location, mechanism, symptoms, and previous occurrences.

In taking the history, you should

1. recall what you saw and heard,
2. talk to the injured player, and
3. talk to other athletes.

If an athlete is unconscious or unable to speak, you will have to rely on what you or the other athletes saw or heard. Also, if you did not see the injury happen, you will have to obtain all of the history from the athlete as well as from other players.

You'll want to find answers to the following questions:

- Was the injury caused by direct contact with another player, equipment, or the ground?
- Was the injury caused by a twisting or turning motion?
- Was there a pop, crack, or other noise when the injury occurred?
- Where does it hurt?
- Did the athlete feel anything unusual when the injury happened? Was there pain, numbness, tingling, weakness, grating, or a snapping feeling?
- Has the athlete suffered this injury before?

Inspection

After you've figured out what's injured and how it happened, you need to **check** the ath-

lete for obvious signs of injury. These include deformities, swelling, skin color changes, consciousness, and other signs. If the athlete is unconscious, start your secondary survey at the head and work down the body. For a conscious athlete, you may begin the survey around the injured area. When you do, look for the following:

1. *Bleeding*—is it profuse or slow? Dark red or bright red?
2. *Skin appearance*—is the skin pale or flushed? Dry or sweaty? Is it blue or gray?
3. *Pupils*—compare the two pupils. Are they dilated (enlarged), constricted (small), or uneven in size? Also, use the penlight from your sport first aid kit and check whether each pupil reacts to light by constricting (see Figure 4.9). If the pupils are uneven or do not react to light, the athlete may be suffering from a head injury.

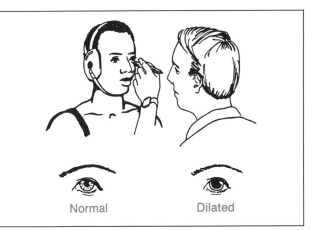

Figure 4.9 Checking pupils.

4. *Deformities*—do you see any indentations, bumps, or other unusual things that shouldn't be there? If a deformity is apparent on an arm or a leg, always compare it to the one on the other side.
5. *Swelling*—is there any puffiness around the injured area?
6. *Discoloration*—is there any bruising or other marks?

Touch

Sometimes, looks can be deceiving. What appears on the surface to be an intact, fully functioning body part may in fact be severely damaged internally. So, to get a better idea of the nature of the injury, **gently** touch the area with your fingertips. When you do, **check** for these conditions:

1. *Point tenderness*—is there an area that is extremely painful?
2. *Skin temperature*—feel the skin with the back of your hand. Is it hot? Cool?
3. *Sensation*—is the area numb?
4. *Deformity*—can you feel any bumps or indentations that you did not see in the inspection?

Take some time now and review the procedures of the secondary survey, shown in Figure 4.10. These techniques are secondary in name only; they are essential first aid measures.

Once you've completed the primary and secondary surveys, you should have a good idea of what's injured and what's wrong with it. Now you need to apply first aid **care** to the athlete. The next chapter will give you some general guidelines to follow.

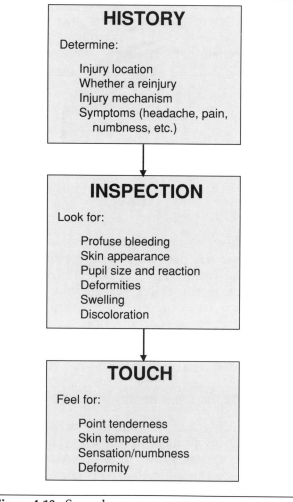

Figure 4.10 Secondary survey summary.

Sport First Aid Recap

1. When an athlete suffers an injury, immediately evaluate his or her safety, position, equipment, and level of consciousness.

2. If unconscious, **call** for emergency medical assistance.

3. Next, begin a primary survey to **check** the athlete's vital signs (ABCs: airway, breathing, and circulation).

4. If the athlete has any breathing or circulation problems, make sure that emergency medical assistance has been **called**, then begin life-saving first aid **care**.

5. If the athlete's heart and breathing rates are normal, begin a secondary survey to pinpoint the site and exact nature of an injury.

6. To do a thorough secondary survey, follow the HIT process: history, inspection, and touch.

7. Once you've determined the location and type of injury, begin administering appropriate first aid **care**.

CHAPTER 5

First Aid Basics

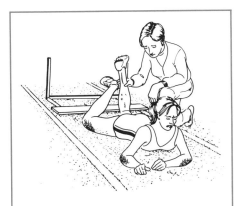

Kathy Allen falls while competing in a 100-meter hurdle race. When Coach Ann Chase reaches her, Kathy is suffering from both cinder abrasions and spike puncture wounds to her legs. Coach Chase wonders if she should treat both types of wound the same. She doesn't realize that these two injuries require slightly different treatments.

To be a truly effective sport first aider, you need to know what emergency treatment is appropriate for each different injury. Although most of the injuries you'll encounter will be superficial cuts, minor contusions, sprains, and strains, you must also be prepared to handle more serious injuries in case they occur.

Before treating any injury, you must get as much information about the injury as you can from the athlete. This means using the HIT (history, inspection, and touch) procedures described in chapter 4.

In obtaining the injury history, you'll listen for the athlete's symptoms or complaints. Symptoms describe how the athlete feels. For example, an athlete may say, ''I feel a grating sensation,'' or ''My knee aches.'' These are symptoms. During your inspection, you'll look for signs of injury. Some common signs of injury that you'll see are swelling, discoloration, and deformity. So, look for signs and symptoms that will help you determine how to administer first aid.

SPORT FIRST AID PRIORITIES

When an athlete is injured, your priorities, in order, should be to

1. initiate your emergency action plan (see chapters 2 through 4),
2. maintain life support,
3. control profuse bleeding,
4. minimize widespread systemic tissue damage,
5. splint unstable injuries,
6. control slow, steady bleeding, and
7. minimize local tissue damage.

Note. If you suspect a head or spine injury, you must immobilize the head and spine before giving any first aid care.

Maintain Life Support

Maintaining the ABCs (airway, breathing, and circulation) is the top priority in first aid care. If in your primary survey you find an athlete is having problems with any of these, immediately send for medical help and begin life-sustaining efforts. Refer to chapter 7 to learn how to provide first aid for choking, breathing difficulties, and circulatory problems. And don't forget your ABCs after you begin administering to the site of injury. You must continually monitor the vital signs of any seriously injured athlete, even though his or her airway, breathing, and circulation may initially be normal.

Control Profuse Bleeding

Check for profuse bleeding after the primary survey, and treat it after you've initiated rescue breathing or CPR, if necessary. If someone is available to assist you, instruct that person in how to administer first aid for profuse bleeding while you administer rescue breathing or CPR.

Anytime a tissue is cut (laceration), punctured, torn (avulsion), bruised (contusion), or scraped (abrasion), it will bleed. This happens most often to the skin, where scrapes, cuts, and bruises are almost an everyday occurrence.

**THE THREE TYPES
OF EXTERNAL BLEEDING**

Arterial
Sign: Rapid, bright red blood flow (may spurt)
Cause: Very deep incision, laceration, or puncture of an artery

Venous
Sign: Rapid, dark blood flow
Cause: A deep incision, avulsion, or puncture of a vein

Capillary
Sign: Slow, oozing blood
Cause: A superficial skin injury such as an abrasion or laceration

---

With open wounds, the threat of disease transmission must be eliminated. So, before administering first aid for bleeding, be sure to protect yourself against exposure to infected blood by wearing effective blood barriers such as disposable surgical gloves or plastic bags on your hands.

Bleeding can also occur internally, from injuries such as bruised muscles, ruptured spleens, and bruised kidneys. Bleeding injuries of the internal organs and how to handle them are explained in chapter 9.

First Aid for Bleeding

Any arterial or uncontrollable venous bleeding is considered life-threatening. If one of your athletes bleeds this severely, immediately take the following actions:

1. Send for medical assistance.
2. Cover the wound with sterile gauze.
3. Apply direct pressure over the wound with your hand. Pressure should be firm and may cause slight discomfort to the athlete.
4. Elevate the injured part (see Figure 5.1).

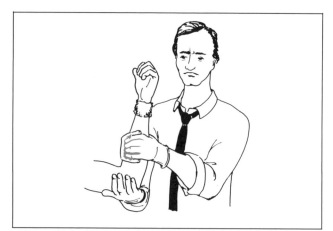

Figure 5.1   Direct pressure and elevation.

5. Monitor the ABCs and perform rescue breathing or CPR, if necessary.
6. Treat for shock, if necessary (see pp. 54-55).

After you've performed the first four steps, the bleeding should stop. But if it doesn't, try to reduce the blood flow by compressing the main artery that supplies blood to the area. These brachial and femoral pressure points are shown in Figures 5.2 and 5.3, respectively.

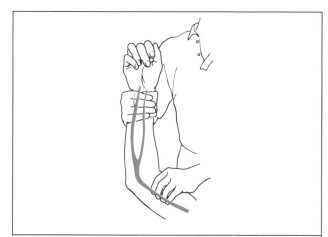

Figure 5.2 Pressure point over brachial artery.

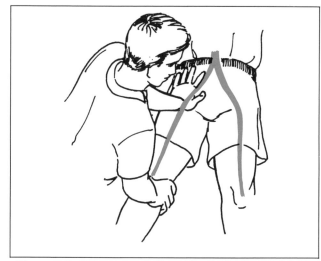

Figure 5.3 Pressure point over femoral artery.

For Bleeding Injuries

DO NOT . . .

. . . attempt to pull out any embedded objects.

. . . remove blood-soaked bandages from a wound. Doing so may cause the bleeding to start again. For example, if you push gauze into a wrestler's nose to stop bleeding, leave the gauze in place until the match is finished.

. . . give aspirin to the athlete. Aspirin can cause increased bleeding.

A Word About Blood-Borne Pathogens

Don't let a fear of human immunodeficiency virus (HIV), hepatitis B, or other blood-borne pathogens keep you from administering first aid to injured athletes. Learn more about these diseases and how they can be transmitted. You can contact your state athletic association for specific sports rules and policies regarding blood-borne pathogens. For example, some sports require athletes to change a bloody uniform before returning to competition.

PRECAUTIONS TO PROTECT AGAINST BLOOD-BORNE PATHOGENS

If your care of an injured athlete involves handling

- bloody wounds or dressings,
- mouth guards,
- body fluids, or
- bloody linen or clothing,

then practice the following guidelines:

1. Wear surgical gloves.
2. Wear safety glasses or a face shield if your face will be exposed to blood or body fluids.
3. Immediately wash your hands after removing the surgical gloves.
4. Immediately wash any skin that comes in contact with blood or body fluid.
5. Place contaminated gloves and bandages in a biohazard waste bag.
6. Clean contaminated floors, equipment, and other surfaces with a 1:10 solution of bleach and water.
7. Use a resuscitation face shield or mask to administer rescue breathing or CPR.
8. Bag contaminated linens or clothing, then wash them in hot water and detergent.

Review your school district's plan for

1. disposal of contaminated waste,
2. handling athletes who are infected with blood-borne pathogens,
3. reporting employees' (coaches', teachers', etc.) exposure to blood-borne pathogens, and
4. protecting employees against the transmission of blood-borne pathogens (i.e., policies, procedures, equipment, and possibly hepatitis B vaccination).

Minimize Systemic Tissue Damage

In the event of injury, illness, or dehydration the body may react by attempting to maintain blood, water, and oxygen supplies to the brain, heart, lungs, and other life-sustaining organs. If the body does react in this way, it deprives other tissues of these same life-sustaining resources. This can result in systemic or widespread tissue damage.

In addition to respiratory and cardiac arrest, three other conditions can lead to systemic tissue damage: shock, heatstroke, and hypothermia.

Treating for Shock

When injured or sick, the body may shut down blood flow and therefore oxygen flow to the extremities and skin in an effort to save the vital organs. Damage can occur if tissues are deprived of blood and oxygen for a long period. This is called shock. If not treated, shock can cause extensive and irreversible tissue damage and even death.

Regardless of the severity of the injury, be alert to any of the signs and symptoms of shock, because shock can occur with minor

as well as serious medical conditions. An injured athlete may be at risk for shock if he or she

- has a low pain tolerance,
- is emotional,
- is tired,
- is dehydrated, or
- is exposed to extreme heat or cold.

First Aid for Shock

History
You may want to consult the athlete's emergency medical card to determine whether the athlete

has a low pain tolerance, or

has suffered previously from shock.

Symptoms
Dizziness and/or nausea

Fatigue and/or weakness

Thirst

Signs
Scared or restless appearance

Weak and rapid pulse

Cool and clammy skin

Sweating

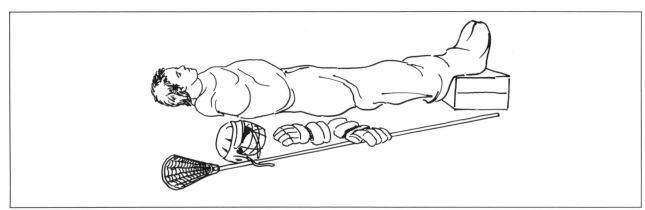

Figure 5.4 Position for a conscious athlete in shock. No suspected head, breathing, or spine problems.

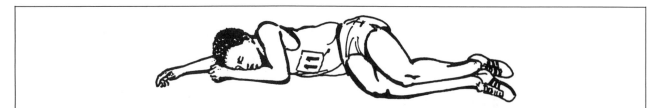

Figure 5.5 Position for an unconscious athlete in shock. No suspected head, breathing, or spine problems.

WHEN TREATING FOR SHOCK

DO NOT . . .

. . . elevate the feet or head of an athlete you suspect has head or spine injuries. Stabilize the head and neck with the athlete lying flat.

. . . give fluids or food to the athlete.

. . . cover an athlete who is already warm.

. . . elevate the feet if the athlete has trouble breathing; elevate the head instead.

Dilated pupils

Shallow and rapid breathing

Shaking or shivering

Pale skin

Bluish lips and fingernails

First Aid

Send for emergency medical assistance.

Position the athlete appropriately.

A conscious athlete with a normal pulse and breathing pattern and no suspected head or spine injury should lie faceup with the feet elevated (see Figure 5.4).

An unconscious athlete with a normal pulse and breathing pattern and no suspected head or spine injuries should lie on the side to allow fluids to drain from the mouth (see Figure 5.5).

An athlete with a possible head or spine injury should lie faceup and flat on the ground.

See chapter 6 for further details on how to move an injured athlete.

Maintain normal body temperature. Don't cover an athlete who is already hot. However, do protect an athlete who is exposed to cold.

Treat for bleeding and other injuries.

Monitor the ABCs and provide rescue breathing or CPR if necessary.

Reassure the athlete.

To decrease the chance of shock occurring, monitor any sick or injured athlete for signs of shock, treat the athlete, and summon medical help immediately.

Heatstroke

In addition to respiratory and cardiac arrest and shock, a loss of body fluids represents a real danger to life-sustaining tissues. If the body does not replenish fluids lost through sweat, dehydration can cause extensive tissue damage. This can also trigger a condition known as heatstroke.

In heatstroke the body reacts to extreme dehydration by shutting down the sweating mechanism to prevent water loss. But sweating is a primary means for the body to cool itself. Robbed of its ability to sweat, the body may continue to rise in temperature, resulting in tissue damage and perhaps even death. If the body temperature reaches 106 degrees or more, the athlete can die if not immediately treated.

Preventing Heatstroke

Dehydration, which can quickly lead to heatstroke is easy to prevent. Give athletes water breaks at least every 20 minutes during activity. Then make sure that they drink at least one cup of water during the break. Also, tell athletes to drink at least two cups of water before practice or games.

Do not allow athletes to wear heavy equipment or vinyl sweatsuits when exercising in hot and humid conditions. The equipment and sweatsuits may hinder the evaporation of sweat—a primary coolant of the body.

Hypothermia

During prolonged exposure to cold temperatures, body tissues are also at risk. As the body's temperature starts to fall, blood is restricted to the vital organs. If the condition persists, widespread tissue damage can occur. Hypothermia can eventually lead to death as cold blood starts to circulate to the brain and heart.

Preventing Hypothermia

Monitor the wind chill and schedule practices indoors if the temperature drops to dangerous levels. Also make sure that athletes wear appropriate protective clothing and that they stay active when practicing or competing in the cold.

For more information on how to evaluate and treat heatstroke and hypothermia, see chapter 11.

Splint Unstable Injuries

Bone fractures, joint dislocations and subluxations, and Grade II and III ligament sprains must be stabilized by splinting to prevent further tissue damage. Here are seven rules for applying splints:

1. *Do not move the athlete until all unstable injuries are splinted.* You should consider moving an athlete only if he or she is in danger of further injury or requires repositioning for rescue breathing, CPR, or control of profuse bleeding or shock.
2. *If emergency medical personnel will arrive within 20 minutes of the injury, let them splint the injury.* Your first aid responsibility is preventing the athlete from moving until emergency medical personnel arrive.
3. *If the arrival of emergency medical help will take longer than 20 minutes, splint the injury in the position in which you found it.* Do not attempt to put fractured or dislocated bones back into place. Repositioning a bone may sever nerves and arteries as well as cause further damage to the bones, ligaments, cartilage, muscles, and tendons.
4. *Cover the ends of exposed bones with sterile gauze.* Do not attempt to push exposed bones back under the skin.
5. *Splint only with rigid or bulky materials that are well padded.* You don't need expensive manufactured splints. Tongue depressors, boards, cardboard, bats, magazines, blankets, and pillows can be used as splints.
6. *Splints should extend to the joints above and below the injury.* For example, for a possible thigh fracture the splint should extend from the hip joint down to the ankle.
7. *Secure the splint.* Place ties above and below the injury, but not directly over it.
8. *Periodically check the skin color, temperature, and sensation of the splinted limb.* Splints that are applied incorrectly or too tightly can compress nerves and arteries. If an athlete complains of numbness or if the skin appears blue or gray or feels cold, then the splint is too tight.

Pages 57 and 58 show proper splinting techniques for the upper arm (Figure 5.6), elbow (Figure 5.7), forearm and wrist (Figure 5.8), finger (5.9), thigh (5.10), kneecap (5.11), lower leg (5.12), and ankle and foot (5.13).

Control Slow, Steady Bleeding

After all the unstable injuries are splinted, you should administer first aid for nonprofuse but steady bleeding. Athletes who suffer superficial skin lacerations or incisions must be treated to stop the bleeding. These types of cuts happen most often to the face, head, arms, and legs.

Treat such injuries the same as you would those involving profuse bleeding. See page 52 for treatment procedures.

If an incision or laceration stops bleeding but is open, apply butterfly strips. Here's how:

1. Gently clean the area around the wound.
2. Apply tape adhesive around the wound with a cotton tip applicator.
3. Pull the butterfly strips from one side, across the wound and to the other side, as shown in Figure 5.14. This will pull the edges of the wound together.
4. Cover with a sterile gauze pad.
5. Send the athlete to a physician.

If you do not have butterfly strips, simply secure the gauze by wrapping over it with roller gauze or elastic wrap. If the bleeding does not stop or if it worsens, send for medical assistance. Continue to apply direct pressure and elevation. And, if necessary, compress the pressure point.

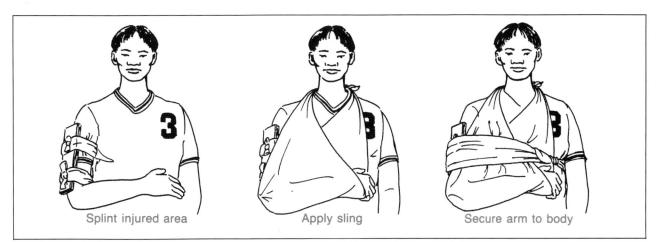

Figure 5.6   Splinting for upper arm injury.

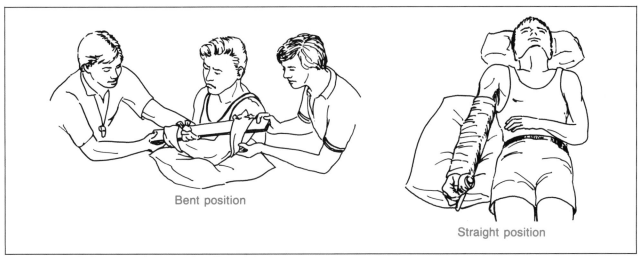

Figure 5.7   Splinting techniques for elbow injuries.

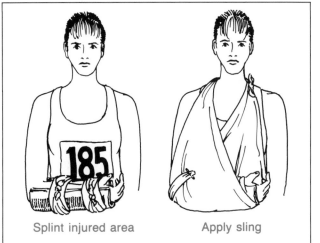

Figure 5.8   Splinting techniques for forearm and wrist injuries.

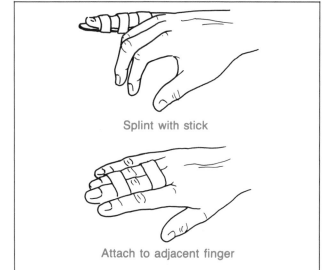

Figure 5.9   Splinting techniques for finger injuries.

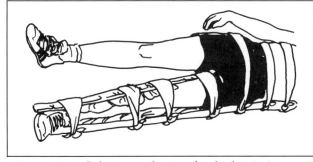

Figure 5.10 Splinting technique for thigh injuries.

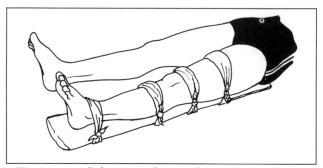

Figure 5.11 Splinting technique for kneecap injuries.

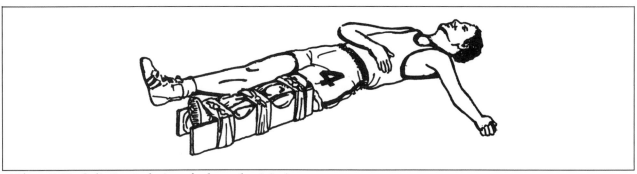

Figure 5.12 Splinting technique for lower leg injuries.

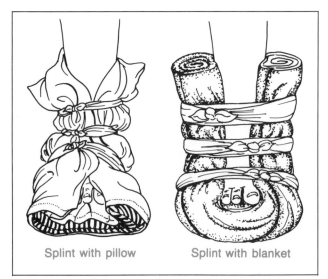

Splint with pillow   Splint with blanket

Figure 5.13 Splinting techniques for ankle and foot injuries.

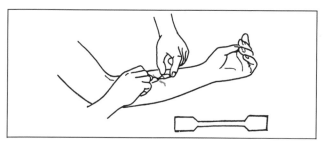

Figure 5.14 Applying butterfly strips.

Minimize Local Tissue Damage

If part of the body is injured, the body's reaction will cause damage to the tissues sur-rounding that part. For example, in an ankle sprain, not only does the injured ligament bleed and swell, but the tissues around it do, too. That's why you see discoloration and swelling all around the ankle joint.

Injury or infection to a particular area can cause any of the following localized tissue reactions:

- Bleeding or loss of fluid
- Swelling
- Temperature increase
- Pain
- Loss of function (inability to use a body part)

PRICE is Right

The best way to prevent these negative local responses is to apply the PRICE principle:

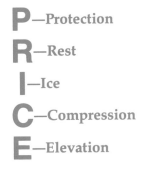

P—Protection

R—Rest

I—Ice

C—Compression

E—Elevation

All of the components of PRICE work to reduce the chance of further injury to the area. In addition, they minimize swelling, which helps prevent further tissue damage.

Protection

We've already talked about protecting fractures, dislocations, sprains, and other unstable injuries by splinting (pages 57 and 58). Additional protective measures include minimizing shock or conditions that can cause further tissue damage. This means protecting the athlete from further injury by not allowing him or her to move around and by keeping other athletes and hazards clear of the athlete.

Rest

An injured athlete should be removed immediately from competition. Do not allow the athlete to return to participation until he or she is examined and released by a physician and is able to play without pain or loss of function (i.e., no limping, no decrease or adjustments in arm movements).

Ice

During the first 24 to 72 hours following an injury, ice can be applied to help minimize pain and control swelling caused by bleeding and fluid loss. Apply ice to the injured area for 15 to 20 minutes. Typically, athletes to whom ice is applied will experience cold, pins and needles, dull aching, and numbness sensations.

Once the area is numb, ice can be removed. It can be applied every two hours as necessary for pain and swelling during the first 24 to 72 hours after an injury.

Crushed ice in a plastic bag works best and can be placed directly over the injury. Water frozen in paper cups can also be used to massage an injured area. Although convenient, commercial ice packs do not stay cold long enough and also may cause skin burns if punctured.

When Applying Ice

DO NOT . . .

. . . apply ice to an athlete who has no feeling in an area or is sensitive to cold. Allergic reactions to ice include blisters, red skin, and rashes.

. . . keep ice in place for more than 20 minutes or apply with a tight compression wrap. Nerve damage may result.

. . . apply ice directly over an open wound.

Compression

To control swelling, you can apply an elastic wrap to an injured limb, especially the foot, ankle, knee, thigh, hand, or elbow. Here are some key steps to follow when applying compression:

1. Start several inches below the injury.
2. Wrap in an upward, overlapping spiral, starting with even and somewhat tight pressure, then gradually wrapping looser above the injury.
3. Periodically check the skin color, temperature, and sensation of the injured area to make sure that the wrap isn't compressing any nerves or arteries.

Elevation

Used in combination with ice and compression, elevation can also help to minimize swelling (see Figure 5.15). The injured part should be elevated above the heart as much as possible for the first 24 to 72 hours following an injury.

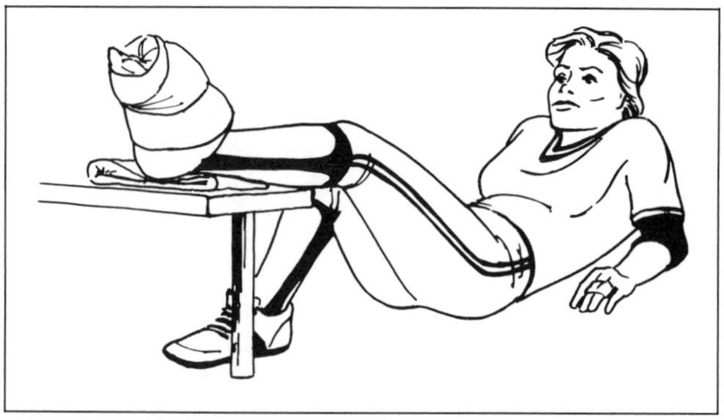

Figure 5.15 Protection, rest, ice, compression, and elevation applied to the ankle.

Sport First Aid Recap

1. When treating an injured athlete, you should first activate your emergency action plan.
2. Treat any breathing and cardiac problems, and immobilize any suspected head or spine injuries.
3. Attempt to stop any profuse bleeding by applying direct pressure, elevation, and digital pressure over the pressure points if necessary.
4. Prevent and treat any systemic tissue damage such as shock or heatstroke.
5. If emergency medical assistance is delayed for more than 20 minutes, immobilize unstable musculoskeletal injuries using well-padded, rigid materials. A splint should extend to the joints above and below the injured area.
6. Try to stop any slow, steady bleeding.
7. Use PRICE (protection, rest, ice, compression, and elevation) to minimize local tissue damage caused by swelling, increases in local tissue temperature, and other reactions to injury.

CHAPTER 6

Moving an Injured Athlete

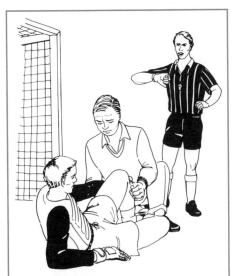

With time ticking down to the last few seconds, the opposing soccer team somehow manages to break away with the ball toward your team's goal. They take what seems to be a sure scoring shot, but your goalie, Ellis Johnson, makes a spectacular dive to prevent the ball from entering the goal. Unfortunately, rather than jumping for joy with his fellow teammates, Ellis is writhing in pain. The referee signals for an injury time-out as the young goaltender lies on the ground; he has an apparent knee injury. You're afraid to move Ellis, but the officials and opposing coach are eager to resume the game. What should you do? Will you risk further injury to Ellis by helping him from the field?

One of the most difficult decisions in giving first aid care is when to move an injured athlete. In this chapter you'll find some general guidelines to consider before making that decision, and you'll also learn how to move athletes with specific types of injuries.

General Rules for Moving

As with all first aid procedures, the basic rule for moving injured athletes is to err on the side of caution. Therefore, move an athlete only if (a) he or she is in danger of further harm, or (b) you are unable to evaluate or treat the injury.

Moving Critically Injured Athletes

For life-threatening or serious injury or illness, keep the athlete still unless you cannot establish an airway or provide rescue breathing or cardiopulmonary resuscitation. Critical conditions include

- respiratory or cardiac arrest;
- head, neck, or back injury;
- shock;
- profuse bleeding;
- internal injuries;
- large joint (ankle, knee, elbow, etc.) dislocations;
- fractures of the ribs, pelvis, shoulder girdle, or long bones (arms and legs); and
- seizures.

It is especially important not to move an unconscious athlete unless it is absolutely necessary. If you must move the athlete to evaluate and treat for respiratory or cardiac arrest, **always** assume the athlete may be suffering from a head or spine injury. Therefore you must completely immobilize the head, neck, and back before moving the athlete.

Moving Noncritically Injured Athletes

Less severely injured athletes can be more readily moved, but you must still exercise extreme caution. If necessary, you may move an athlete suffering from these conditions:

- Grade I sprain and strain (see page 38)
- Solar plexus injury ("wind knocked out")
- Contusions
- Facial injuries
- Closed finger, hand, and wrist fractures
- Finger dislocations

When Moving Noncritically Injured Athletes

DO NOT . . .

. . . attempt to move the athlete from the playing area until all unstable injuries are immobilized or splinted, or until the athlete regains composure and is able to walk with assistance from the field.

Proper Moving Techniques

Just as your sport has certain skills that enhance performance and increase safety, so too does sport first aid. When you must move an athlete or are asked to assist emergency medical personnel, you should be prepared to use the most sound and safe techniques for moving. Depending on the situation, these are the skills you and the rest of your coaching staff should know:

- Three- or four-person rescue
- One-person rescue
- One-person walking assist
- Two-person walking assist
- Four-handed carrying assist
- Two-handed carrying assist

Three- or Four-Person Rescue

This technique is commonly used to place an unconscious or seriously injured athlete on his or her back, for example, on a spine (back) board or stretcher. First, check the ABCs or administer lifesaving first aid to an unconscious athlete. Then, to place the athlete on the spine board, an emergency medical technician or trained first aider should go to the athlete's head and direct the other rescuers. This lead person must follow these steps:

1. Grasp the head, holding onto both sides of the head and jaw. A neck collar should be placed on the athlete if one is available.
2. Command the other rescuers to position themselves at the shoulder, hips, and legs, as shown in Figure 6.1a.
3. Instruct another individual to place the spine board next to the athlete.
4. On the count of three, instruct everyone to roll the athlete (who would be facing away from the board) as a unit (see Figure 6.1b).
5. Slide the board next to the athlete's back.
6. Slowly lower the athlete onto the board.

One-Person Rescue

If you have no qualified assistance, do not move the unconscious athlete unless rescue breathing or cardiopulmonary resuscitation is required. If you must move the athlete yourself, do the following:

1. Position yourself behind the athlete, near the head and shoulders.
2. Place the athlete's arms and legs close to the body, if possible (see Figure 6.2a).
3. Cradle the head with one hand to help stabilize the neck (see Figure 6.2b). It is important to cradle the head and move the athlete as a unit to help prevent aggravating any spine injuries.
4. Place your other hand on the athlete's shoulder and roll his or her body, as a unit, toward yourself.
5. Position the athlete as comfortably as possible with a minimum of movement (see Figure 6.2c).

The use of four-, three-, and one-person rescues is necessary only for critical injuries, and when the athlete is unconscious. We hope that you'll only rarely encounter such critical con-

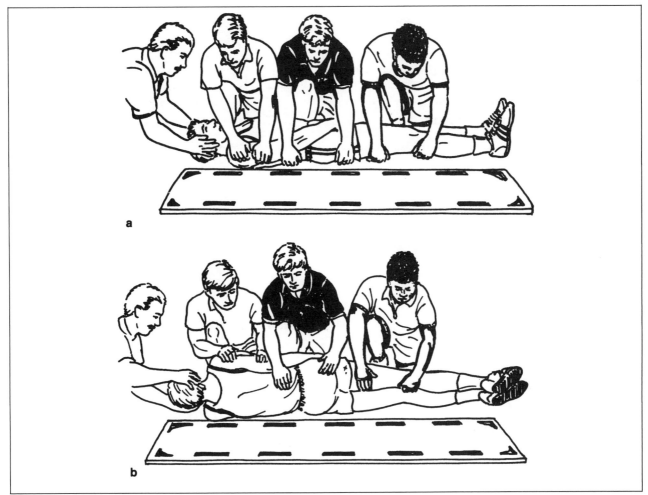

Figure 6.1   Four-person rescue: (a) preroll positions, (b) roll body as unit.

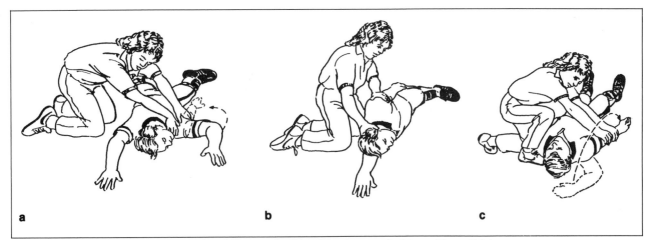

Figure 6.2   One-person rescue: (a) stabilize neck, (b) roll body as unit, (c) position athlete.

ditions. More commonly, you'll face situations in which an athlete has a minor or moderate injury such as a muscle pull or arm contusion. When this type of situation arises, use the following moving techniques.

One-Person Walking Assist

This assist is ideal for walking a dazed or slightly injured athlete off the playing area by yourself. Here's how to do it:

1. Place the athlete's arm around your shoulder, and hold his or her hand close to your chest.

2. Grasp the athlete around the waist with your free hand.

3. Instruct the athlete to lean on you as needed when walking (see Figure 6.3).

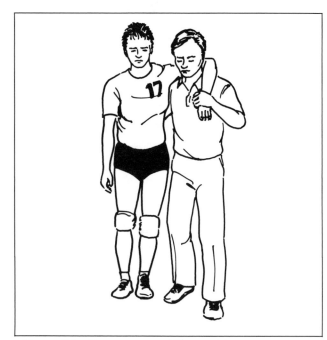

Figure 6.3   One-person walking assist.

Two-Person Walking Assist

If someone else is available to help you, it is better to use the two-person walking assist. However, be certain that the assistant will follow your directions, so as not to endanger the well-being of the athlete. Here's a step-by-step list of instructions to give your helper:

1. "Stand on the opposite side of the athlete from me."

2. "Place the athlete's nearest arm around your shoulder and hold on to the hand."

3. "Grab the athlete around the waist."

4. "Slowly walk to the sidelines, supporting the athlete with your arms and shoulders" (see Figure 6.4).

Four-Handed Carrying Assist

If an athlete has an injured leg but is able to assist you in moving himself or herself, then

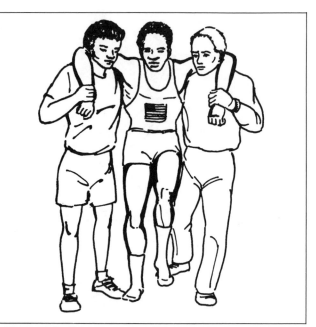

Figure 6.4   Two-person walking assist.

To Protect Yourself

DO NOT . . .

. . .attempt the following assists if you have a history of back or leg problems or if you are considerably smaller than the athlete.

---

use the four-handed carry. This carry is especially useful if it is too far or too difficult for the athlete to move with the two-person walking assist.

To perform this assist, recruit a helper who is willing to take and obey the orders you give. Instruct the helper as follows:

1. "Grasp your right forearm with your left hand."

2. "Hold on to my left forearm with your right hand." Meanwhile, grip your own right forearm with your left hand, and then grasp your helper's left forearm with your right hand (see Figure 6.5a).

3. Instruct the athlete to sit on your arms and place his or her arms around you and your assistant's shoulders (see Figure 6.5b).

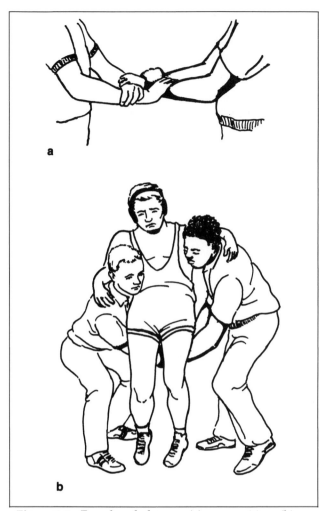

Figure 6.5 Four-handed carry: (a) arm position, (b) carry technique.

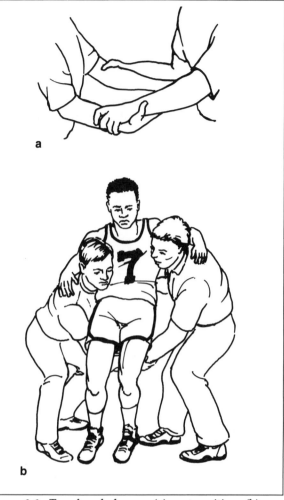

Figure 6.6 Two-handed carry: (a) arm position, (b) carry technique.

Two-Handed Carrying Assist

At times, a player may suffer foot injury that precludes any weight bearing activity. In such cases, the two-handed carrying assist is the best option for moving the athlete. Also, use this assist to carry an athlete who is unable to walk with assistance. To correctly perform this carry, you and an assistant should do the following:

1. Grasp each other's forearms (see Figure 6.6a).
2. Instruct the athlete to sit on your and your assistant's nearest arms and put his or her arms around your shoulders.
3. Support the athlete's back with your free arms (see Figure 6.6b).
4. Slowly lift the athlete by straightening your legs.

Sport First Aid Recap

1. Seriously injured athletes should almost never be moved.

2. The only times that you would ever move a seriously injured athlete are when he or she is in a position that prohibits you from evaluating the ABCs, prevents you from administering life-saving first aid, or poses significant danger of causing the athlete further injury from the environment.

3. If an unconscious athlete or an athlete you suspect has head, neck, or back injuries must be moved, always stabilize the head and spine first and move the body as a unit. Do not let the body twist when it moves.

4. Athletes with fractures, dislocations, subluxations, or Grade II or III strains or sprains should not be moved until the injuries are splinted or immobilized.

PART III

Sport First Aid for Specific Injuries

Now that you are familiar with your sports medicine teammates, your first aid responsibilities, basic anatomy, and evaluation and first aid procedures, you may want to review what you've learned. The information presented in the first six chapters is a lot to absorb, but it's essential that you know those basics before you proceed to the next eight chapters. After all, you wouldn't expect your athletes to run a play in a game situation without reviewing it in practice. So, if you have any doubts about your understanding of the information in chapters 1 through 6, review that section of the book.

If you're confident about your comprehension of that material, you are ready to learn how to apply it to specific injury situations. This next section is similar to the game-situation drills that your athletes perform in practice. You'll learn what common signs and symptoms to look for when evaluating certain sport injuries. And you'll learn how to administer first aid for these injuries.

The chapters in Part III proceed from life-threatening injuries to minor problems. Although it's unlikely that you'll have to evaluate and treat a life-threatening situation during your coaching career, it's vital that you learn how to do it; your athletes' lives depend on it. Chapters 7 through 11 will familiarize you with potential life-threatening problems such as respiratory and cardiac arrest, head and spine injuries, internal organ injuries, sudden illnesses, and temperature-related illnesses. Ligament sprains, muscle strains, joint dislocations, contusions, and abrasions are more common injuries that athletes suffer. These types of injuries are covered extensively in chapters 12 through 14.

By no means will the chapters in this section teach you all you need to know about evaluating and treating specific sport injuries. In fact, it is essential that you get CPR training through the Red Cross or other certifying agency. These chapters will, however, direct you in how to properly act in the event of a certain type of injury situation; and as a coach, who so often is the initial care giver, you owe it to your athletes to be prepared to help them when they need it.

CHAPTER 7

Respiratory and Circulatory Emergencies

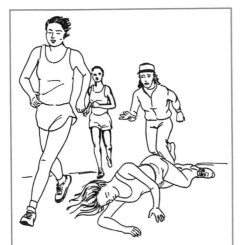

Your third-best runner is running the race of her life. She knows the team's counting on her to finish in the top 25 to qualify the school for the state meet. Her gutsy performance comes to an abrupt halt as she collapses a half mile from the finish line. As you rush to her side, you see that she is having trouble breathing, and her face is changing color. What do you do?

You learned the ABCs when you were young. But do you remember the ABCs of sport first aid—airway, breathing, and circulation? They are the first three things you should check in your primary survey of an injured athlete. So if you have any doubts about them, review chapter 4.

The ABCs are extremely important to know because (a) the body cannot survive very long without oxygen; (b) when breathing stops, the heart and brain are affected (brain tissue death can occur in as little as 5 minutes); and (c) when the heart and brain stop functioning, life ends.

This chapter will help you determine if an athlete is having problems with breathing or circulation and what you can do to help. Of course, you must know the basics of sport first aid described and illustrated in Part II of this book. And you must send someone for help, reminding the caller to tell the emergency medical personnel that it is a life-threatening injury. Then you must immediately begin emergency first aid **care**.

Specifically, these circulorespiratory conditions require emergency first aid:

Airway obstruction—a conscious or unconscious athlete is choking.

Respiratory arrest—an athlete is unconscious and not breathing.

Cardiac arrest—an athlete is unconscious and not breathing, and the heart is not beating.

The remainder of this chapter covers these three conditions sequentially. Additionally, within the analysis of each condition, we've indicated the various degrees of severity to which an athlete may experience the problem. By examining these different respiratory and cardiovascular problems, you'll be better prepared to evaluate and provide emergency care should any of your athletes suffer from these conditions.

Sport First Aid for Airway Obstruction

Figure 7.1 is a flowchart of the first aid procedures for treating airway obstruction in both conscious and unconscious victims. It also covers what to do for a partial obstruction as

well as a total obstruction. Review the chart carefully, then continue reading about the specific obstruction first aid techniques.

Partial Airway Obstruction in a Conscious Athlete

Suppose that an athlete runs off the field in a panic. She is grasping her throat and making high-pitched gasping noises. What should you do?

1. First ask, "Are you okay?" If she says "yes," but has trouble breathing or

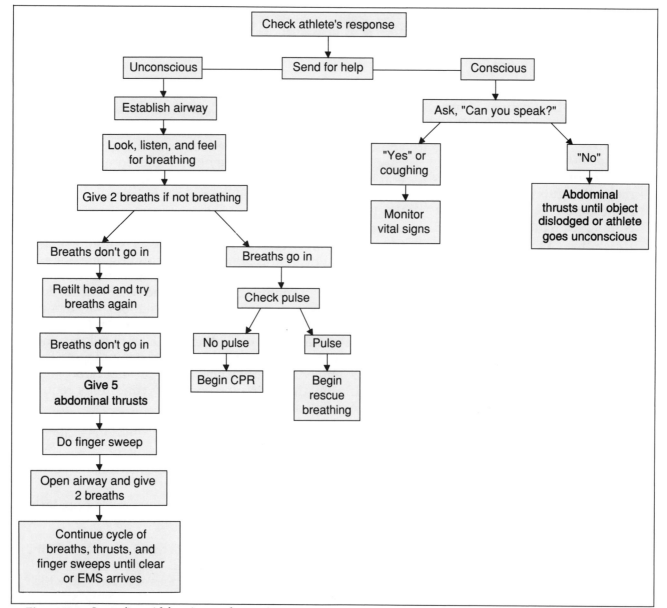

Figure 7.1 Sport first aid for airway obstruction.

grasps her throat (the universal choking sign), she may have a partially blocked airway.

2. Encourage her to cough.
3. Monitor the athlete until (a) the object is dislodged and she breathes normally, or (b) her airway is totally obstructed. If this happens, perform the Heimlich maneuver described in the next section.
4. Send the athlete to a physician.

For Partial Airway Obstruction

DO NOT . . .

. . . slap an athlete on the back if his or her airway is partially blocked. This may loosen the object and cause it to totally block the airway.

Total Airway Obstruction in a Conscious Athlete

Now suppose that the athlete cannot cough and is only making high-pitched wheezing noises. The first thing to do is ask, ''Can you speak?'' If she shakes her head ''no,'' or gives the universal choking signal, you should immediately begin first aid for choking—the Heimlich maneuver.

Heimlich Maneuver

The Heimlich maneuver was introduced in the early 1970s as a first aid technique for complete airway obstruction. It is widely used today and is taught as part of CPR classes by both the American Red Cross and the American Heart Association.

The technique uses compressions to force air out of the lungs and dislodge the obstruction. It has been found to be highly effective if performed correctly.

Performing the Heimlich maneuver
1. Stand behind the athlete.
2. Place your foot between the athlete's feet.
3. Wrap your arms under the athlete's armpits and around the waist, just above the navel.
4. Make a fist with your hand and place your thumb and index finger just above the athlete's navel (see Figure 7.2).

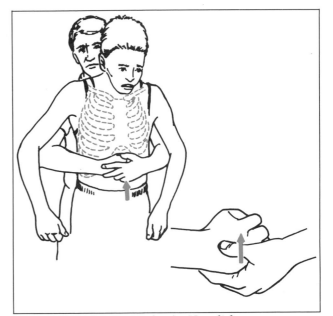

Figure 7.2   Positioning for the Heimlich maneuver.

5. Grab your fist with your other hand.
6. Thrust inward and upward against the athlete's diaphragm (located just above the stomach).

When Performing the Heimlich Maneuver

DO NOT . . .

. . . place your fist too high, covering the tip of the breastbone. The thrusts could break the tip of the breastbone and cause internal injuries.

If the athlete can speak or cough, stop doing the Heimlich maneuver and encourage the athlete to cough. Otherwise, keep doing the Heimlich compressions one at a time until you dislodge the object or the athlete loses consciousness.

Airway Obstruction in the Unconscious Athlete

What if you are not able to dislodge the object and the athlete loses consciousness? Don't panic! In fact, the object will be easier to remove because the athlete's muscles will become totally relaxed.

If an athlete loses consciousness from choking, you should do the following:

1. Protect the athlete from injury. If you've been performing the Heimlich maneuver while standing, support the athlete with your leg and body and slowly lower him or her to the floor.

2. Place the athlete on his or her back (see chapter 6).

3. Open the athlete's mouth by placing your thumb in the athlete's mouth and hooking it under the lower teeth. Grasp the chin with your fingers and gently lift the chin up.

4. Using your other hand, sweep your index finger with a hooking motion through the athlete's mouth (see Figure 7.3). Start along the opposite cheek, move across the back of the tongue, then along the cheek nearest you.

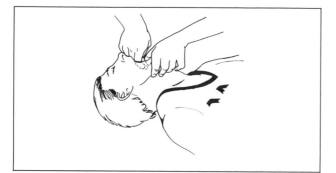

Figure 7.3 Performing a finger sweep.

5. Establish an airway with either the head tilt/chin lift or chin lift only (for suspected head and spine injuries).

6. Attempt to give two breaths from the position shown in Figure 7.4.

7. If your breath does not go in and make the chest rise, perform 5 consecutive abdomi-

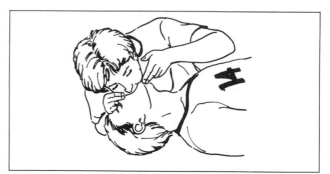

Figure 7.4 Positioning for breaths.

nal thrusts with the heel of your hand. Position yourself by straddling the athlete's thighs and placing the heel of your hand between the athlete's navel and breastbone. Your fingers should be pointing toward the head. Place your other hand on top and thrust upward toward the chest (see Figure 7.5).

Continue this cycle until the object becomes dislodged and you are able to check for breathing and circulation. Perform a primary survey (see pages 44-48) as you would if one of your athletes was unconscious and you did not see how the injury occurred.

If the athlete is not breathing and/or does not have a pulse, you will have to start either rescue breathing or CPR. If the athlete is breathing, monitor the breathing and pulse rates, and treat for shock if necessary, until medical assistance arrives.

If you come upon an unconscious athlete and your primary survey shows an obstructed airway, you should do the following:

1. Send someone to get emergency help.
2. Perform 5 manual thrusts to either ab-

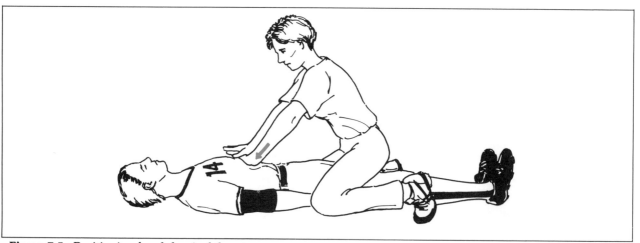

Figure 7.5 Positioning for abdominal thrusts.

domen or, if you suspect internal injuries, to the chest at hte middle of the breastbone.

3. Perform a finger sweep.
4. Attempt to give two breaths.

Continue this cycle until the object is dislodged.

5. If the object dislodges, check breathing and pulse.

Airway obstruction is a life-threatening condition; its treatment cannot be left to chance. Therefore, be prepared to apply the techniques described here if you are called upon to save a choking athlete's life.

Sport First Aid for Respiratory Arrest

Let's assume that you've gone out to help an athlete who is not breathing. You've performed a primary survey for airway, breathing, and circulation. And you've established that the athlete has a pulse but is not breathing. The next step is to begin rescue breathing.

Before you learn rescue breathing techniques, however, examine the respiratory arrest first aid flowchart in Figure 7.6. It outlines the steps that you will take in the event of a respiratory emergency.

You may also want to review how to perform the primary survey, described in chapter 4. This survey should be your initial first aid measure in the treatment of a respiratory arrest.

Rescue Breathing

Rescue breathing is a technique used to supply air to an individual who is not breathing. If you blow air into an athlete's lungs, that air contains enough oxygen to help sustain his or her life.

So if an athlete is not breathing but has a pulse, you should follow these steps.

1. Send someone to get emergency help.
2. Maintain an open airway with the head tilt/chin lift or chin lift only.
3. Place a CPR mask over the athlete's nose and mouth.

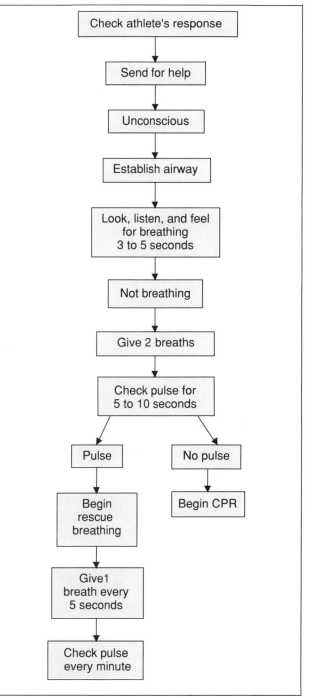

Figure 7.6 Respiratory arrest sport first aid.

4. If the mask does not fully envelop the nose and mouth, pinch the nose shut.
5. Seal your mouth over the athlete's mouth (see Figure 7.7).
6. Blow in one full breath.
7. Turn your head to the side to watch the athlete's chest fall and hear and feel the breath being exhaled (see Figure 7.8).
8. While watching the chest, count "1 one thousand, 2 one thousand, 3 one thousand,"

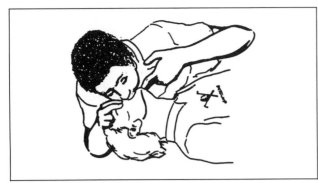

Figure 7.7 Position for rescue breathing.

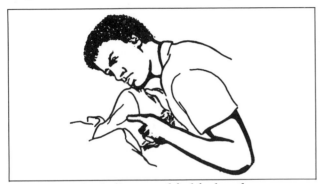

Figure 7.8 Look, listen, and feel for breaths.

breathe in at "4 one thousand," then give one slow, full breath at "5 one thousand."

9. Continue with this pattern of providing a breath every 5 seconds.

10. Check the pulse after 1 minute, then periodically every 1 to 2 minutes thereafter. Remember, you must check the pulse for at least 5 seconds.

With an unconscious athlete who has an obstructed airway, you may need to administer rescue breathing once the object is dislodged. However, once it is dislodged, be sure to check to see if the athlete is able to breathe on his or her own before you initiate rescue breathing. If he or she is still not breathing, begin rescue breathing.

Continue rescue breathing until

- the athlete begins to breathe,
- the rescue team takes over, or
- the athlete's heart stops beating (cardiac arrest), when you should begin cardiopulmonary resuscitation.

Sport First Aid for Cardiac Arrest

Cardiac arrest occurs when an athlete stops breathing and his or her heart stops beating.

If quick first aid intervention is not begun within 6 minutes of the onset of cardiac arrest, permanent brain damage will result and the athlete will likely die. Although fatalities and catastrophic injuries average 36 occurrences a year for all high school sport programs in the United States (NATA, 1989b), these emergencies require quick initiation of cardiopulmonary resuscitation (CPR) to save an athlete's life. The late U.S. Olympic volleyball athlete Flo Hyman and Loyola Marymount basketball player Hank Gathers were two of the more publicized cases of cardiac arrest in sport.

Cardiopulmonary resuscitation is a first aid technique involving both rescue breathing and heart (chest) compressions. The theory behind CPR is to artificially supply oxygen to the athlete with rescue breathing and pump the heart by compressing the chest. The American Red Cross and the American Heart Association offer certification in CPR. You should obtain certification from one of these organizations so that you are current with the latest CPR techniques.

Now, suppose that you came upon an athlete who was not breathing and did not have a pulse. What would you do? Begin cardiopulmonary resuscitation. The steps to take are illustrated in Figure 7.9.

Cardiopulmonary Resuscitation

CPR has three components: positioning, compression, and breathing techniques. Each of these techniques must be performed effectively for CPR to work. In addition, you must know how to properly cycle the use of these CPR skills during the precious seconds you have to revive an athlete. The list that follows explains precisely how you should position yourself and the athlete, apply breaths and compressions, and cycle the use of the techniques in giving CPR:

Positioning
1. Position the athlete faceup on a hard surface.
2. Kneel next to the athlete's side.
3. Using your hand that's closest to the athlete's waist, run your index and middle fingers along the inside of the athlete's ribs up toward the chest until you feel the tip of the xiphoid process (lower edge of the breastbone).

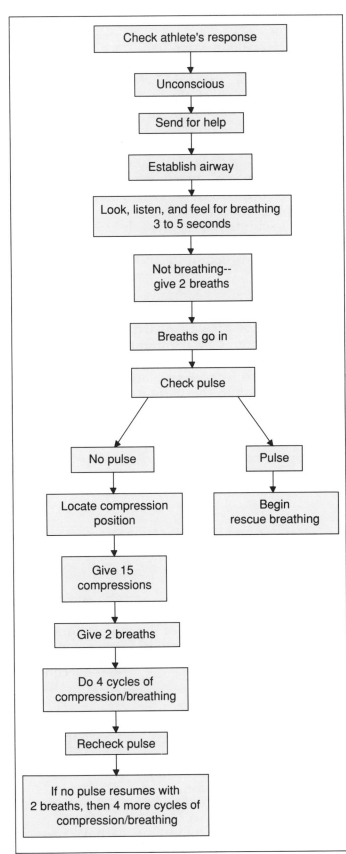

Figure 7.9 CPR sport first aid.

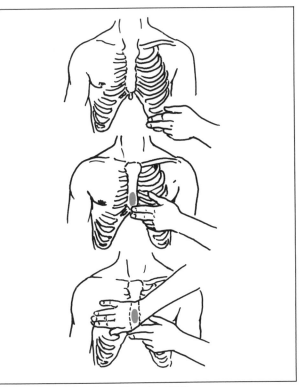

Figure 7.10 Hand position for CPR.

4. Rest your fingertips on the top of the xiphoid process, and place the heel of your free hand next to your index finger (see Figure 7.10).

5. Your fingers should be pointing across the chest and away from your body.

6. Place your other hand on top of the hand resting on the chest.

7. Straighten your fingers and then interlock them by bringing the fingers of the top hand down through the spaces between the fingers of the bottom hand.

8. Allow only the heel of your hand to touch the athlete's breastbone. Don't let your fingers touch the ribs.

9. Straighten your elbows and position yourself so your shoulders are directly over your hands, as shown in Figure 7.11.

Compression and Breathing

10. Push straight down against the chest with the heels of your hands (see Figure 7.12).

11. For adults, compress the chest only 1-1/2 to 2 inches and no further. For children 8 years and younger (not infants), compress the chest 1 to 1-1/2 inches with one hand only.

12. In adults, deliver 15 compressions in a

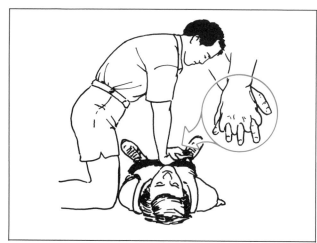

Figure 7.11 Body position for CPR.

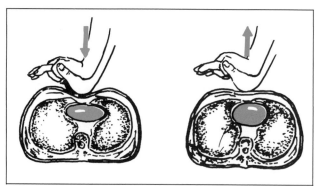

Figure 7.12 CPR chest compressions.

row using the sequence, ''1 and 2 and 3 and 4 and 5 and . . . '' up to 15 (the rate of 80 to 100 compressions per minute).

13. After the 15th compression, go back to the head, open the airway, close off the nose, seal your mouth over the athlete's mouth, and blow in two breaths (see Figure 7.13).

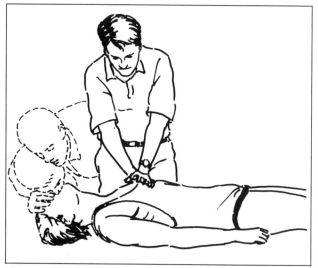

Figure 7.13 CPR compression and breathing sequence.

Cycling
14. Reposition your hands for CPR and perform 15 chest compressions again.

15. Do four cycles of 15 compressions/two breaths, then check the pulse (pulse should be checked approximately every 2 minutes).

16. If there is no pulse, give two breaths, then 15 compressions.

17. Use this cycle of 15 compressions/two breaths until the athlete begins to breathe and the heart starts to beat, or until emergency help takes over.

18. In children the CPR cycle is 5 compressions/one breath (use one hand). During compressions count, "1 and 2 and 3 and 4 and 5."

Remember, this chapter presents only an overview of airway obstruction, rescue breathing, and CPR techniques. **It does not replace certification through the Red Cross or American Heart Association.**

In addition to these life-threatening conditions, your athletes may experience any one of several other life-threatening respiratory problems. Let's take a quick look at how to apply first aid for these conditions.

Additional Respiratory Difficulties

Sickness, allergic reactions, anxiety, and contact injuries can also cause breathing problems in athletes. Some of the more common breathing problems in athletes are caused by the following:

- Near drowning
- Anaphylactic shock
- Asthma
- Collapsed lung
- Bruised throat
- Pneumonia or bronchitis
- Solar plexus spasm
- Hyperventilation

You'll learn how to evaluate each of these conditions, listen and look for specific symptoms, and look for specific signs. Then you'll learn how to administer first aid for each injury. The more serious or life-threatening conditions are presented first, followed by the more common, less serious breathing problems.

Near Drowning

Definition
The athlete breathes water into the lungs, which blocks the transfer of oxygen to the blood.

History
Ask the athlete, ''Are you choking?''

The athlete responds by shaking his or her head ''yes.''

Sign
The athlete is coughing or using the universal choking sign (grasping the throat).

First Aid
If the athlete is coughing, don't attempt first aid; simply monitor him or her.

If the athlete is unable to speak or cough or is unconscious, begin the Heimlich maneuver and rescue breathing or CPR.

Send for medical assistance, and continue first aid until medical help arrives.

Be sure the athlete is examined by a physician.

Playing Status
The athlete cannot return to activity until he or she is released by a physician.

Prevention
Supervise athletes closely while they are in the water.

Forbid horseplay around a swimming or diving area.

Anaphylactic Shock

Definition
This is a condition in which an athlete has an allergic reaction to a substance. The body responds with swelling in the throat area, which narrows the air passages.

Causes
Allergic reactions to insect stings, certain types of food, mold, and other substances. See chapter 10 for more information.

History
Ask ''Were you stung by a bug?'' ''Did you eat or come in contact with a substance that you are allergic to?''

Symptoms
Tightness in the chest

Inability to breathe

Signs
The athlete makes wheezing or gasping noises.

Skin, fingernails, or lips may appear blue or gray.

First Aid
Send for medical assistance.

Apply ice to the area.

Monitor the ABCs and provide rescue breathing or CPR if necessary.

Playing Status
The athlete cannot return to activity until he or she is released by a physician.

Prevention
Check the playing area for insect nests.

Know the medical history of any athlete with allergies.

Asthma

Definition
This is a condition in which the air passages in the lungs constrict and therefore interfere with normal breathing.

Causes
Allergic reaction to dust or molds

Exposure to cold environments such as ice skating rinks

Exposure to smoke or other inhaled substances

Adverse response to strenuous exercise

Symptoms
Tightness in the chest

Inability to breathe

History
Ask athlete, ''Do you have asthma?''

Signs
The athlete has trouble exhaling.

The athlete makes wheezing noises when breathing.

Fingernails, lips, or skin may turn blue or gray.

Pulse rate may increase to 120 beats per minute or more.

The athlete is noticeably frightened.

Reassure the athlete.

Place the athlete in a comfortable position.

Ask, "Do you have any asthma medication with you?"

Assist the athlete with the asthma medication.

Monitor the athlete's breathing, pulse rate, and skin color.

Send for emergency medical assistance if the athlete does not improve.

Begin rescue breathing or CPR if necessary.

Playing Status
The athlete cannot return to activity until he or she is released by a physician.

Prevention
Be aware of all your athletes who have asthma.

Encourage asthmatic athletes to take an active role in managing their condition.

Remind them to bring their medication to all practices and games.

Monitor asthmatic athletes who compete in cold or dusty environments.

Give the athletes with asthma frequent rests during activity.

Collapsed Lung

Definition
The lung partially collapses due to air or fluid pressure (see Figure 7.14).

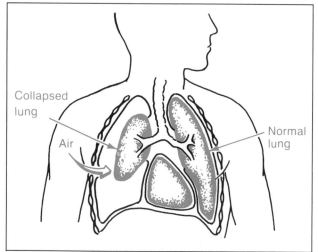

Figure 7.14   Collapsed lung.

Causes
The athlete experiences a direct blow to the ribs that compresses or tears the lung.

Spontaneous collapse of a lung, not caused by an injury.

The lung is punctured by a sharp object such as broken ribs, an arrow, or a javelin. (Note: A collapsed lung can also be punctured by a broken rib caused by incorrect chest compressions in CPR.)

History
Recall how the injury happened.

Ask the athlete, "Where does it hurt?"

If no injury occurred, question the athlete about a history of respiratory problems.

Symptoms
Inability to breathe

Chest pain

Signs
Bruise or open wound in the chest

Sucking noise coming from an open chest wound

The athlete may be gasping for air

Increased breathing rate

First Aid
Send for emergency medical assistance.

Reassure the athlete.

Place the athlete in a comfortable position.

Cover any open, sucking wound with a non-porous material such as aluminum foil or extra thicknesses of sterile gauze.

Monitor the ABCs and provide rescue breathing and CPR if necessary.

Playing Status
The athlete cannot return to activity until he or she is released by a physician.

Prevention
Forbid horseplay.

Enforce safety regulations during archery or javelin practice or competition.

Bruised Throat

Definition
This is a contusion to the throat, through which air passes to the lungs.

Causes

The athlete experiences a direct blow to the throat area. This happens most often when an athlete gets hit with a baseball, softball, or hockey puck. A bruised throat can also be caused by a direct hit from an elbow in basketball or football.

History

Athlete is hit in the throat by an object.

Symptoms

Pain in the throat

Inability to breathe

Signs

The athlete may be gasping for air.

His or her breathing rate may increase.

There is swelling or discoloration where the object hit the throat.

Some deformity in the throat area may be apparent.

The area may make a crunchy or grating sound when touched.

First Aid

Reassure the athlete.

Place the athlete in a comfortable position.

Apply ice to the injured area to help reduce swelling (see chapter 5 for more details on the use of ice).

Monitor the ABCs and provide rescue breathing or CPR if necessary.

Send for medical assistance if the athlete does not improve.

Treat for shock if necessary (see chapter 5).

Playing Status

The athlete may return to activity if breathing and pulse return to normal and he or she has no pain or deformity in the throat area.

Prevention

Require all field hockey, lacrosse, and ice hockey goalies and baseball and softball catchers to wear throat protectors.

Pneumonia or Bronchitis

Definition

An inflammation or infection of the lungs caused by a virus or other microorganism. These conditions can cause fluid or mucus to collect in the lungs.

Causes

Infection by a microorganism

Irritation by an inhaled substance such as dust or chemicals

History

Possible fever

Coughing

Possible chronic respiratory problems (asthma, bronchitis, etc.)

Symptoms

Shortness of breath

Tightness in the chest

Signs

Possibly a fever

Labored breathing

Coughing, possibly with mucus

First Aid

Make the athlete comfortable.

Send the athlete to a physician.

Playing Status

The athlete cannot return to activity until he or she is released by a physician.

Prevention

Do not let an athlete participate until he or she has fully recovered from a respiratory infection.

Solar Plexus Spasm

Definition

The solar plexus is a nervous system structure located just below the rib cage (see Figure 7.15). This condition is commonly described as a person's "having the wind knocked out" of him or her.

Cause

Direct hit to the area

Symptoms

Inability to breathe in, or inhale

Pain just below the breastbone

Signs

Possibly temporary unconsciousness

Labored breathing or hyperventilation

First Aid

Reassure the athlete.

Loosen constricting clothing.

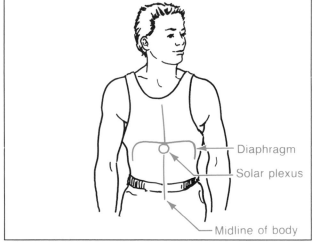

Figure 7.15 Solar plexus.

Encourage the athlete to relax.

Instruct the athlete to take a short breath followed by a slow, deep breath.

Monitor the ABCs.

Complications
If the athlete does not recover within a few minutes, suspect other injuries and take the following actions:

Send for emergency medical assistance.

Check for other injuries and treat them.

Monitor the ABCs and provide rescue breathing or CPR if necessary.

Playing Status
The athlete can return to activity if breathing and pulse return to normal and the athlete has no deformity and no more pain in the area.

Prevention
Be sure athletes wear required or recommended protective padding. This is especially important in football and hockey.

Hyperventilation

Definition
In this condition, the athlete breathes rapidly and deeply. This creates a deficit of carbon dioxide in the bloodstream and upsets the oxygen and carbon dioxide balance.

Causes
The athlete becomes excited and starts breathing deeply and rapidly.

A blow to the solar plexus.

Symptoms
Inability to breathe

Tingling in the arms or hands

Dizziness or light-headedness

Panic or anxious feeling

Signs
Rapid and deep breathing

Pulse rate increases

If the athlete doesn't recover, the nailbeds or lips may turn blue or gray.

First Aid
Reassure the athlete.

Place the athlete in a comfortable position.

As a last resort, instruct the athlete to place a paper bag or hand over his or her nose and mouth and breathe into it until the symptoms subside.

Complications
If the athlete does not recover within a few minutes, take the following actions:

Monitor the ABCs and provide rescue breathing or CPR if necessary.

Send for emergency medical assistance.

Check for other injuries that could be contributing to the problem.

Playing Status
The athlete may return to activity once breathing and pulse return to normal. Be sure to continually check the athlete for signs of recurrence.

Prevention
Try to calm an excitable athlete.

Teach anxious or excitable athletes correct breathing techniques.

Sport First Aid Recap

1. Although uncommon, circulatory and respiratory problems can be life-threatening, and therefore they demand prompt and appropriate first aid.

2. An obstructed airway cuts off the flow of oxygen to the body and must therefore be treated with the Heimlich maneuver.

3. Correct technique for the Heimlich maneuver with a conscious athlete involves administering abdominal thrusts with your fist between the athlete's navel and breastbone. Thrusts are continued until the object is dislodged.

4. Do not attempt the Heimlich maneuver on an athlete with a partially obstructed airway; simply encourage the athlete to cough.

5. For an unconscious victim with an obstructed airway, administer a cycle of finger sweeps of the athlete's mouth, two breath attempts, and 5 abdominal thrusts until the object is dislodged.

6. Rescue breathing is a technique of blowing in air to supply oxygen to an athlete who is not breathing.

7. The correct rate of breaths for secondary schoolers and adults is one breath every 5 seconds. (For children, the correct breathing rate is one breath every 3 seconds.)

8. Cardiopulmonary resuscitation is used for athletes who are in cardiac arrest. It involves providing oxygen to the athlete via rescue breathing and pumping the heart with chest compressions.

9. The correct sequence and rate of CPR compressions and breaths is 15 compressions to two breaths for adults at a rate of 80 to 100 compressions a minute. The cycle for children is 5 compressions and one breath.

10. Near drowning, anaphylactic shock, asthma, collapsed lung, throat contusions, and pneumonia and bronchitis are other potentially life-threatening breathing and respiratory problems.

11. Solar plexus spasms ("wind knocked out") and hyperventilation are more common and less serious breathing problems that athletes suffer.

CHAPTER 8

Head and Spine Injuries

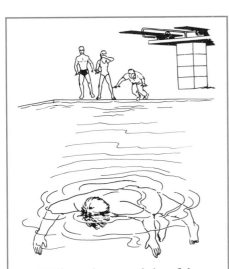

Joe Wilson is practicing his dives off the 3-meter board for the conference meet. As Joe leaps off the board and is rotating backward, his head strikes the board. He limply falls into the pool and slowly floats to the surface. Realizing that Joe is unconscious, Coach Eckert dives into the pool to rescue Joe. How should Coach Eckert move Joe and administer first aid?

We've all seen head and spine injuries in sport, especially in contact sports such as football and wrestling. But they also occur in diving, basketball, baseball and softball, and soccer. The following scenarios are all too familiar:

Dazed boxers staggering in a struggle to remain standing

Confused football players wandering off the field to the wrong sidelines

Soccer players crumbling to the ground after a collision

Basketball players crashing helplessly to the floor after their feet are cut out from under them

What should you do if an athlete stumbles off the field in a stupor or is knocked unconscious? This chapter will tell you.

Head Injuries

First of all, we need to define what constitutes a head injury. For our purpose, it is an injury to the brain tissue or skull. Four types of injuries fit this definition:

- *Concussion*—a temporary malfunction of the brain that involves actual brain damage
- *Contusion*—bleeding and possibly swelling of the brain tissues
- *Hemorrhage and hematoma*—bleeding or pooling of blood between the tissue layers covering the brain or within the brain
- *Fracture*—a crack or break in the skull

When administering to an athlete with a head injury, don't get hung up on trying to decide which type of head injury he or she has suffered. All are caused by similar mechanisms and all have similar symptoms and signs. If you suspect a head injury, concentrate your efforts on treating it. And always assume a concomitant spine injury has occurred as well.

For Head Injuries

DO NOT . . .

. . . remove an athlete's helmet until you've ruled out a spine injury.

. . . try to revive an athlete or clear an athlete's head by using smelling salts or ammonia. The strong smell may make the athlete jerk his or her head.

Causes of Head Injuries

Nearly all head injuries are caused by a direct blow. The blow can cause either a skull injury at the point of contact (see Figure 8.1) or a soft-tissue (brain and its covering) injury on the side opposite where the blow occurred (see Figure 8.2). Head injuries can also occur if the head is forcefully and quickly moved, such as in a whiplash-type injury.

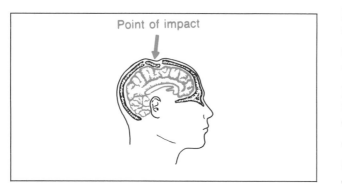

Figure 8.1 Skull injury from a direct blow.

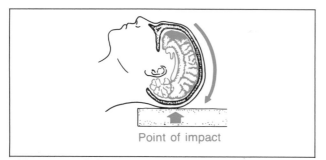

Figure 8.2 Soft-tissue injury on opposite side of direct blow.

First Aid for Head Injuries

Now that you know the types of head injuries that can occur and their causes, let's see what can be done to treat them. The manner in which you apply first aid to an athlete will depend on whether the player is conscious or unconscious.

Conscious Athlete With Head Injury

Evaluation
In your evaluation of a conscious athlete, the mechanism of injury and the athlete's actions are keys to determining the nature and extent of the injury.

History
The athlete received a direct blow or jarring injury to the head.

Symptoms
Dizziness

Ringing in the ears

Headache

Nausea

Signs
Blood or clear fluid is draining from the athlete's nose, mouth, or ears.

There is a bump or deformity at the point of the blow.

Blurred vision.

There is bleeding or a wound at the point of the blow.

The athlete's pupils are unequal in size or display an inappropriate response to light (may not constrict when subjected to light).

The athlete seems confused, disoriented.

The athlete is having convulsions or seizures (see chapter 10).

The athlete experiences a loss of balance.

The athlete's speech is slurred.

There are breathing or pulse irregularities.

The athlete experiences loss of memory—determine recall by asking specific questions such as "What's your phone number? What day is it? Who are we playing?"

The eyes do not track a moving object, such as your finger, as a unit. For example, one eye may be slower in moving than the other.

First Aid
Send for medical assistance. Severe symptoms

such as extended memory loss, slurred speech, seizures, and breathing irregularities indicate a more severe head injury. These injuries require that you call for immediate notification of emergency medical personnel.

Stabilize the head and neck.

Monitor the ABCs and provide rescue breathing or CPR if necessary.

Treat for shock.

Playing Status
The athlete cannot return to activity until he or she is released by a physician. Even when the injury is not severe, the athlete must be monitored in case his or her condition becomes serious. Therefore, an athlete with a minor head injury must be evaluated by a physician.

Prevention
Warn athletes against using their heads as a point of contact if possible.

Make sure all football, hockey, baseball, softball, and lacrosse athletes wear appropriately fitted helmets.

Unconscious Athlete With Head Injury

History
The athlete received a direct blow or jarring injury to the head.

Signs
Unconsciousness

Possibly breathing irregularity or respiratory arrest

Possibly leaking of blood or clear fluid from the mouth, nose, or ears

Possibly pulse irregularities

Pupils may be unequal in size or fail to react to light

First Aid
Send for emergency medical assistance.

Stabilize the athlete's head and neck.

Monitor the ABCs and provide rescue breathing or CPR if necessary.

Control any profuse bleeding.

Treat for shock.

Immobilize any fractures or unstable injuries.

Assist emergency medical personnel with boarding the athlete if necessary.

Playing Status
The athlete cannot return to activity until he or she is released by a physician.

Prevention
Prohibit players from spear tackling with their heads.

Check the fit and condition of all athletes' helmets.

Now that you're familiar with the signs, symptoms, and treatment of head injuries in both conscious and unconscious athletes, let's move on to evaluating and treating spine injuries. In many cases, because of their structural and functional interconnections, an injury to the head will cause damage to some portion of the spine, and vice versa.

Spine Injuries

As we discussed in chapter 3, the spinal column is a system of bones or vertebrae that protect the spinal cord (nerves). The vertebrae are held together by ligaments and muscles. Nerves branch out of the spinal column between the vertebrae (see Figure 3.6).

The spinal column is divided into five sections (see Figure 8.3):

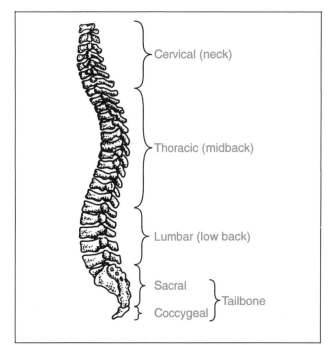

Figure 8.3 Five sections of spinal column.

Any injury to the spinal column can injure the spinal cord, including specific nerve branches. This could result in loss of feeling or sensation and/or paralysis—loss of temporary or permanent function in certain body parts.

Types of Spine Injuries

The most common spine injuries in sport are sprains, fractures, contusions, and strains. Each can result in serious injury to the spinal cord.

- *Sprain*—if any of the spinal ligaments are stretched or torn, the stability of the spinal column is affected. This would allow the vertebrae to shift on top of each other and possibly pinch or injure a nerve or the spinal cord.
- *Fracture*—a broken vertebrae can pinch a nerve or injure the spinal cord.
- *Contusion*—a bruise to the bone, muscle, or spinal tissue can cause bleeding and swelling, which in turn can constrict or pinch the spinal cord or nerves.
- *Strain*—any stretching or tearing injuries of the muscles and/or tendons can also affect the stability of the spinal column.

Causes of Spine Injuries

Because the spinal column is the hub around which all body movement occurs, you will want to protect athletes against such injuries with proper equipment and techniques. Even so, the spinal column can be injured by the following:

- *Direct blow*—usually causes fractures and contusions (see Figure 8.4)
- *Compression*—often results in fractures, contusions, and sprains (see Figure 8.5)
- *Torsion or twisting*—may cause fractures, sprains, and strains (see Figure 8.6)

Evaluation of Spine Injuries

Regardless of the type, mechanism, and site of the injury, your evaluation of a suspected spinal injury should be conducted in the same manner. And, because it is very diffi-

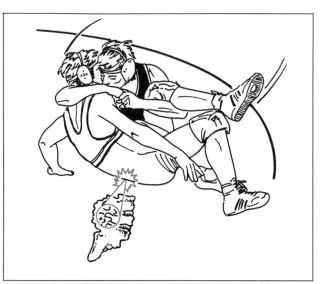

Figure 8.4   Direct blow injury.

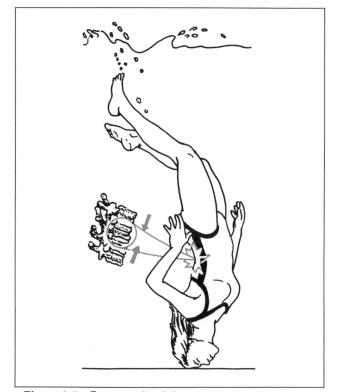

Figure 8.5   Compression injury.

cult to differentiate between a sprain, fracture, contusion, and strain, the treatment you apply should be the same for all. Always suspect a serious head and/or spine injury in an unconscious athlete. Never move the athlete during the evaluation unless you are unable to check the ABCs or unless the athlete is in danger of further injury.

If an athlete walks off the playing area and complains of pain anywhere along the spine,

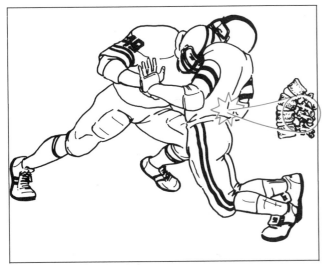

Figure 8.6 Torsion injury.

perform the evaluation with the athlete in the position in which you initially see him or her. For example, a standing athlete should remain standing. Also, if an athlete is wearing a helmet, leave it on! Removing it can cause further harm. If you suspect a serious head or spine injury, immediately stabilize the head and spine and treat the athlete for shock and other injuries as necessary.

**STEPS IN EVALUATING
FOR SPINE INJURY**

Check for the following:

1. Response or consciousness
2. The ABCs (airway, breathing, and circulation)—particularly in an unconscious athlete; provide rescue breathing and CPR if necessary
3. Profuse bleeding—both internal and external
4. Shock
5. Neurological damage—numbness and tingling first, followed by an inability to move the fingers or toes, then weakened grip strength (see under Symptoms and Signs)
6. Fractures, dislocations, sprains, strains, and so on
7. Slow bleeding wounds

Spine Injury

History
The athlete suffered a direct blow, compression, or torsion injury to the spine.

Symptoms
Numbness or tingling in the toes, feet, fingers, or hands

You can easily check these by asking the athlete to name the finger or toe that you are touching.

Pain on or near the spine

Signs
Inability to move the fingers or toes

Grossly unequal hand grip strength. Have the athlete try to squeeze your fingers.

Muscle spasms near the spine

Possibly breathing difficulties

First Aid
Send for emergency medical assistance.

Immobilize the athlete's head and spine.

Provide rescue breathing or CPR if necessary in an unconscious athlete. (Use chin lift method only!!)

Treat any profuse breathing.

Treat for shock as necessary.

Treat for any profuse bleeding.

Monitor the pulse and heart rate.

Stabilize any other fractures, dislocations, sprains, or strains.

Playing Status
Any athlete you suspect has a head or spine injury should be evaluated and released by a physician before returning to activity. This is true with even minor injuries, because they can easily lead to more serious problems.

Prevention
Recommend that all football players who are prone to neck injuries wear neck rolls (see Figure 8.7).

Require all football players and other contact sport athletes to perform neck strengthening after practice. When strengthening the neck, though, do not use neck bridges or rotations.

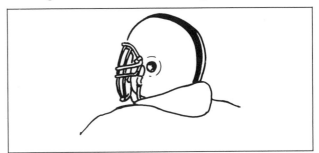

Figure 8.7 Neck roll.

Noncritical Spine Injuries

In addition to serious spine injuries, other less severe nerve problems can occur in sport. The most common of these is a burner or stinger, technically called a nerve impingement.

Burner or Stinger

Definition
A neck burner is a stinging or shocking sensation felt in the back of the neck or shoulder.

Cause
A nerve to the neck or shoulder is pinched by either the bones, muscles, or other neck tissues. This most often occurs when the head is turned quickly to one side and tilted down, as in Figure 8.8.

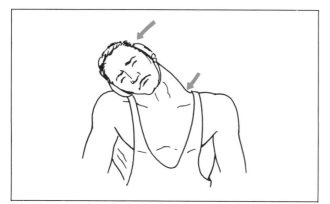

Figure 8.8 Mechanism of a burner injury.

History
Athlete may have suffered a torsion injury to the neck.

Symptoms
Numbness, tingling, or burning in the neck, shoulder, or arm

Feeling of being shocked or struck by a lightning bolt

Signs
Loss of sensation in the arm and/or hand on the injured side

Slight weakness of the arm and/or hand on the injured side

First Aid
Immobilize the head and spine if sensation and strength do not return within 5 minutes.

Monitor the ABCs and provide rescue breathing or CPR if nessessary.

Stabilize any other injuries.

Treat for shock if neccessary.

Refer the athlete to a physician.

Playing Status
The athlete may return to participation if feeling and strength return within 5 minutes and the athlete has no pain or signs of other injuries. However, even athletes with a temporary neck burner should be seen by a physician following the practice or game and before the next practice or game. Athletes who suffer repeated burners or stingers may be disqualified from contact sports, because permanent nerve damage can result.

Prevention
Recommend that all football players who are prone to burners wear neck rolls.

Require neck strengthening for all football players and other contact sport athletes.

Sport First Aid Recap

1. Any head or spine injury can lead to respiratory or cardiac arrest and therefore must be evaluated quickly and treated correctly.

2. Any suspected head and spine injuries must be immobilized not only before you move an athlete, but also before you administer rescue breathing or CPR (utilize chin lift only method).

3. All head and spine injuries should be examined by a physician before the athlete is allowed to return to participation. This

includes even minor back or neck pain and headaches caused by a direct blow, compression, or torsion.

4. Common symptoms of head injuries include dizziness, ringing in the ears, headache, and nausea.

5. Signs of head injury include blood or fluid draining from the nose, mouth, or ears; unequal pupil reaction to light; confusion; seizures; loss of balance; slurred speech; blurred vision; and memory loss.

6. An athlete with a head injury should be removed from activity and monitored for life-threatening conditions and shock.

7. Evaluate and treat an unconscious head-injured athlete by assuming that his or her spine may also be injured. You should therefore immobilize the head and spine.

8. Common symptoms of spine injury include numbness or tingling in the extremities and pain on or near the spine.

9. Loss of function in the arms and legs, unequal handgrip strength, and muscle spasms are common spine injury signs.

10. Burners and stingers refer to injuries in which the nerve(s) to the arm are suddenly pinched in the neck.

11. If numbness or tingling in the arm caused by a burner lasts for more than 5 minutes, immobilize the athlete's head and neck and send for medical assistance.

12. An easy way to help prevent neck burners is to require athletes to strengthen their necks before and throughout the season.

CHAPTER 9

Internal Organ Injuries

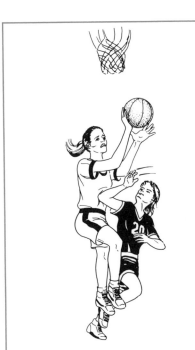

While reaching high to rebound a ball, center Kristie Lane is accidentally hit just below the breastbone by another player also going up for the rebound. Kristie is able to return to the game after sitting out a few minutes. When the game is over, Kristie complains of some abdominal muscle cramps but otherwise feels all right. Later that night, Kristie collapses and goes into shock. At the hospital, her doctor discovers that the blow to the stomach caused her spleen to rupture. He immediately operates on Kristie to stop the internal bleeding.

Although internal injuries are not common in sport, it is vital that they be evaluated properly and treated promptly and correctly. The delicate internal organs are especially vulnerable to contusions. The ribs and pelvis help to protect these areas; however, a direct blow to the wrong spot can cause damage and bleeding.

Internal injuries must be handled by medical personnel, but you can help minimize complications that may arise from them. In this chapter you'll learn how to quickly evaluate internal injuries, alert medical personnel, and monitor the athlete until medical help arrives.

For Suspected Internal Injuries

DO NOT . . .

. . . give an athlete food or water.

. . . allow an injured athlete to leave a game or practice while unattended.

. . . allow an athlete who has suffered an apparently minor blow in the area of an internal organ to go home until you warn both the athlete and his or her parents of the signs and symptoms of a serious internal injury.

It often takes a few hours for a serious internal injury to appear. Therefore, it is essential that an injured athlete be monitored, in case his or her condition worsens.

To ensure proper supervision, give the athlete's parents a card explaining the signs and symptoms of serious internal injuries. The card should also instruct them to immediately take their child to the hospital emergency room if the signs and symptoms of a more serious injury appear (see Figure 9.1).

INTERNAL INJURY INSTRUCTIONS

Call a physician or be assisted to the Emergency Room at a local hospital if your child experiences one or more of the following:

1. Nausea
2. Vomiting
3. Abdominal cramps or rigidity
4. Skin pallor, weak pulse, or dizziness (shock)
5. Discoloration of urine (copper or red)

Figure 9.1 Instruction card for athletes' parents.

Serious Internal Injuries

These are the most common serious internal injuries in sport:

- Ruptured spleen
- Bruised kidney
- Testicular trauma

The next few pages will outline the immediate steps you should take when an athlete suffers any of these three conditions.

Ruptured Spleen

Definition
This is a life-threatening contusion injury to the spleen (see Figure 9.2).

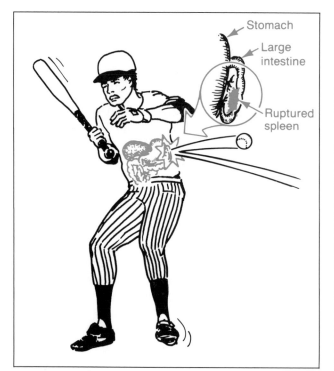

Figure 9.2 Spleen injury.

Cause
The spleen, located on the left side of the body underneath the stomach and lower ribs, is usually injured by a direct blow to either of those areas. The blow bruises the spleen tissue and can cause profuse internal bleeding, because the spleen acts as a reservoir for red blood cells.

History
The athlete received a direct blow to the left upper abdominal area.

Symptoms
Initially, the athlete feels pain in the left upper abdominal area.

Later, pain progresses to the left shoulder and/or neck (as shown in Figure 9.3).

The athlete feels faint or dizzy.

Signs
Initially, tenderness over left upper abdominal area

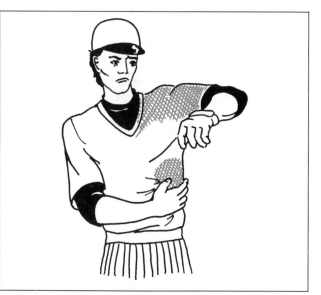

Figure 9.3 Referred pain from a spleen injury.

Abrasion or bruise over injured area

In advanced stages, pale skin, rapid pulse, possibly vomiting, rigid abdominal muscles, low blood pressure, shortness of breath

First Aid

Send for emergency medical assistance if the initial symptoms and signs last longer than a few minutes or progress to the advanced stages.

Monitor the athlete's ABCs and provide rescue breathing or CPR if necessary.

Treat for shock if necessary.

Treat other injuries, such as possible rib fractures.

Playing Status

The athlete cannot return to activity until he or she is released by a physician.

Even if an athlete's signs and symptoms do not progress to the advanced stages, a bruised spleen can easily be ruptured if the athlete returns to participation before the bruise fully heals.

Prevention

Require athletes to wear proper protective padding.

Do not allow athletes suffering from mononucleosis to participate in sport until released by a physician. In mono, the spleen enlarges and is vulnerable to contusion injuries.

Bruised Kidney

Definition

This is a contusion to the kidney (see Figure 9.4).

Cause

Direct blow to either side of the midback

History

The athlete received a direct blow to either side of the midback.

Symptoms

Initially, the athlete feels pain at the site of the blow.

Later, pain moves to the low back, outside thighs, or front pelvic area (see Figure 9.5).

The athlete feels faint or dizzy.

Signs

Bruise or abrasion over the injured area

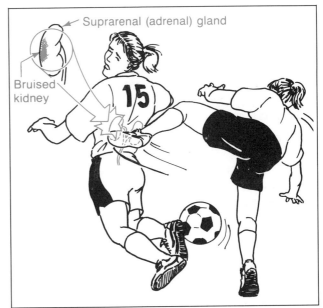

Figure 9.4 Kidney injury.

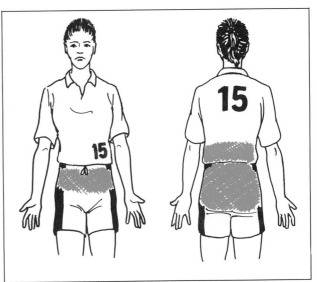

Figure 9.5 Referred pain areas after kidney injury.

Tenderness over the injured area

Frequent and burning urination

Cloudy or bloody urine

Rigid back muscles over the injury site

Pale skin

First Aid

Send for emergency medical assistance if the initial signs and symptoms do not stop within a few minutes or if they progress to the advanced stages.

Monitor the ABCs and provide rescue breathing or CPR if necessary.

Treat for shock if necessary.

Treat other injuries as needed.

Playing Status
The athlete cannot return to activity until he or she is released by a physician. A mildly bruised kidney can worsen over time and become life-threatening.

Prevention
Require athletes to wear proper protective padding such as kidney pads or flak jacket (especially in football).

Testicular Trauma

Definition
This is a contusion or trauma to the testicles.

Cause
A direct blow to the groin area

History
The athlete suffered a direct blow to the groin area.

Symptoms
Pain

Nausea

Signs
Have the athlete perform a self-exam, looking for swelling, discoloration, and deformity.

Spasm

First Aid
Place the athlete on his back.

Push his knees up toward his chest; continue until the pain decreases.

Apply ice for 15 minutes to the area.

Send the athlete to a physician if the pain does not stop after 20 minutes, if the testicles draw upward, or if the athlete has bloody or cloudy urine.

Playing Status
The athlete cannot return to activity until the pain and swelling subside or until he is released by a physician.

Prevention
Require male athletes in contact sports to wear protective athletic supporters, and recommend that they wear cups.

Minor Internal Injuries

Not every internal injury is life-threatening. The most common minor internal injuries are the side stitch and gastritis. The symptoms and signs of these conditions may mock those of a more serious injury. Therefore, do not take even apparently minor injuries lightly.

It is important to conduct a thorough evaluation to determine whether the athlete has suffered an injurious blow. This would indicate a potentially more serious injury. If the athlete was not injured by a blow and began experiencing pain for no apparent reason, then further evaluation is necessary. You'll want to determine whether the athlete has a fever, indicating a possible serious infection. If all else fails and the pain does not subside within a few minutes, send the athlete to a physician or medical facility.

Now let's take a look at a common minor internal injury in sport—the side stitch.

Side Stitch

Definition
This is a cramping feeling felt in either the right or left side. It's most often felt by runners or athletes who lack cardiovascular endurance.

Cause
Unknown

Symptoms
Sharp pain is felt in the side during activity.

The pain usually disappears after the athlete rests.

Signs
None

First Aid
Tell the athlete to bend over and push his or her fingertips into the painful side.

Have the athlete take a deep breath and blow it out through tight lips.

Instruct the athlete to stretch the muscles by placing the arm overhead and bending at the waist over to the opposite side.

Playing Status

The athlete can return to activity once the pain subsides and breathing and heart rates are normal. If the pain does not subside, the athlete must be seen and released by a physician to rule out other problems.

Prevention

Have athletes warm up adequately with light jogging and stretching before strenuous activity.

Instruct athletes not to eat within 2 hours before strenuous activity.

Sport First Aid Recap

1. A direct blow to any of the internal organs can cause serious bleeding injuries.

2. Ruptured spleen, bruised kidneys, and testicular trauma are the serious internal injuries most common in sport.

3. Even if an athlete's pain subsides and the symptoms and signs are minor, monitor the athlete to make sure that the condition doesn't worsen. This includes warning the athlete's parents of the signs and symptoms of a more serious internal injury.

4. Signs and symptoms of a life-threatening internal injury include extreme tenderness, muscle spasm, shock, vomiting, and bloody urine.

5. The side stitch is a common internal organ problem in athletics, although its cause is unknown. Stretching, direct pressure, and deep breathing seem to help decrease the pain.

CHAPTER 10

Sudden Illness

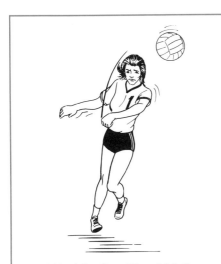

Middle blocker Terri Nelson has been slow to react during the volleyball team's entire practice. Consequently, she is repeatedly hounded by Coach Malone. As the team scrimmages, Terri completely misses a serve, and the ball drops to the floor. Staring blankly at the floor, Terri staggers two steps, then collapses. After Terri regains consciousness, she tells Coach Malone that she has had the flu for the past 3 days. She is running a slight fever and hasn't been able to eat without getting sick.

The seemingly immediate onset of illness can happen to anyone. But all too often, athletes continue to play while sick and attempt to hide their illness from the coach. That does no one any good—particularly the suffering athlete. So ask your athletes to report, and be alert to, common illnesses such as the flu, heat exhaustion, and these other types of sudden illness that strike athletes:

- Diabetic complications
- Drug overdose
- Seizures
- Fainting
- Severe allergic reactions

As a coach, you must be able to quickly recognize the signs and symptoms of these sudden illnesses and administer first aid to prevent them from becoming life-threatening.

Diabetes

Diabetes is a condition that affects the body's ability to properly produce and regulate insulin. Insulin is produced in the pancreas and controls the uptake of glucose (sugar) by body tissues. Glucose is the primary energy source for tissues, especially the brain and kidneys. Without proper insulin levels, the tissues can receive either too much glucose (hyperglycemia) or not enough (hypoglycemia).

Individuals with serious diabetic problems may need to take insulin injections. Because exercise and diet can affect the amount of insulin the body needs, diabetic athletes should be closely monitored for signs of diabetic illness. An athlete who is having problems regulating his or her diabetes will be prone to either insulin shock or diabetic coma. This section explains appropriate first aid measures for diabetes-related conditions.

Insulin Shock

Definition
This is a condition that causes an athlete's glucose (sugar) levels to suddenly drop (hypoglycemia).

Cause
High insulin levels

History
The athlete is a diabetic. (You'll know this by checking the athlete's medical history or medical alert tag.)

Symptoms
Dizziness

Headache

Hunger

Weakness

Signs
Perspiration

Pale and cold skin

Rapid pulse

Drooling

Confusion or disorientation that may progress to unconsciousness

Shock

Poor coordination

First Aid
Send for emergency medical assistance if the athlete does not recover within a few minutes.

Monitor the athlete's ABCs and provide rescue breathing or CPR if necessary.

Treat for shock if necessary.

Give sugar—candy, pop, or fruit juice to a conscious athlete, and granulated sugar or liquid glucose (athlete may carry it) under the tongue of an unconscious athlete.

Playing Status
The athlete cannot return to activity until the insulin level is stabilized. It's best to rest the athlete from all activity for the remainder of the day.

Prevention
Carefully monitor a diabetic athlete during practice and competitions. This may include the use of a predetermined hand signal by the athlete when he or she is not feeling well.

Suggest that the athlete bring fruit juice or candy bars to practice and games.

Diabetic Coma

Definition
In this condition, an athlete suffers from a high blood glucose (sugar) level (hyperglycemia). The body tries to compensate by eliminating excess sugar in the urine. This causes increased urination and therefore dehydration.

Causes
Low insulin level

History
Athlete is a diabetic. (You'll know this by checking the athlete's medical history or medical alert tag.)

Symptoms
Excessive thirst

Dry mouth

Headaches

Abdominal pain

Nausea

Signs
Dry, red, and warm skin

Weak, rapid pulse

Heavy breathing

Excessive urination

Possibly vomiting

Sweet, fruity-smelling breath

First Aid
Send for emergency medical assistance.

Monitor the ABCs and provide rescue breathing or CPR if necessary.

Treat for shock if necessary.

Lay an unconscious athlete on his or her side to allow vomit or fluids to drain from the mouth.

Playing Status
The athlete cannot return to activity until he or she is examined and released by a physician.

Prevention
Make sure the athlete takes frequent water breaks during practice and competitions.

Do not allow an athlete with uncontrolled diabetes to participate.

Drug Overdose

Drug overdose is another possible cause of sudden illness in an athlete. There are two basic categories of drugs:

Depressants—common depressants include alcohol, narcotics (morphine, heroin, and codeine), and barbiturates (phenobarbital). These drugs depress the nervous system. Athletes abuse these drugs typically to achieve a relaxed, calm feeling.

Stimulants—cocaine and amphetamines are the most common. These drugs stimulate the nervous system and make athletes feel quicker and more alert for a period of time.

You should be able to recognize the signs and symptoms of possible overdose of both types of drugs. Moreover, educate and counsel your athletes so you won't have to take the following first aid measures.

Overdose of Depressants

Symptoms
Relaxed feeling

Fatigue

Signs
Pale, cold, and clammy skin

Constricted pupils that may not respond to light

Rapid and weak pulse

Possibly unconsciousness

Shallow breathing that may stop

First Aid
Send for emergency medical assistance if necessary.

Monitor the athlete's ABCs and provide rescue breathing or CPR if necessary.

Lay an unconscious athlete on his or her side to allow fluids or vomit to drain from the mouth.

Treat for shock if necessary.

Speak to the parents or guardian, and send the athlete to a physician if he or she recovers quickly from the overdose.

Playing Status
The athlete cannot return to activity until he or she is examined and released by a physician.

Prevention
Provide drug abuse education for athletes.

Monitor athletes who exhibit these behaviors characteristic of depressant abuse: lethargy, inattentiveness, mood changes, fatigue, and slowed reactions.

Overdose of Stimulants

Symptoms
Lack of fatigue

Irritability

Confusion

Mood changes

Signs
Dilated pupils

Rapid pulse

Hallucinations

Possibly cardiac arrest in extreme cases

First Aid
Send for emergency medical assistance if the symptoms don't improve or if the athlete goes into respiratory or cardiac arrest.

Monitor the ABCs and provide rescue breathing or CPR if necessary.

Lay an unconscious athlete on his or her side to allow fluids or vomit to drain from the mouth.

Treat for shock if necessary.

Speak to the parents and send the athlete to a physician if he or she recovers quickly from the overdose.

Playing Status
The athlete cannot return to play until he or she is examined and released by a physician.

Prevention
Provide drug abuse education for athletes.

Monitor any athletes who exhibit these behaviors of stimulant abuse: hyperactivity or extreme fatigue, mood changes, dramatic changes in performance, and aggressiveness.

Other Acute Illnesses

Seizures, fainting, and anaphylactic shock are other possible sudden illnesses that you may have to face. Epileptic individuals are most prone to seizures, but seizures can also occur in athletes who are suffering from a head injury or dehydration. Fainting in athletes is most often caused by an illness or dehydration. Anaphylactic shock may occur in athletes who are allergic to certain insect stings. Each of these acute illnesses requires quick and accurate assessment and first aid intervention. Let's take a look at each.

Seizures

Definition
A seizure is an abnormal, excessive electrical discharge from the brain cells. It can lead to sudden changes in an athlete's alertness, behavior, and muscle control.

Causes
Because seizures can be caused by a wide variety of problems, it's important to look for other health problems when evaluating an athlete who has just suffered a seizure. Epilepsy is a primary cause of most seizures. Some of the other causes include head injuries, brain infections, respiratory arrest, high fevers, and heatstroke.

History
The athlete has a history of epilepsy. (You'll know this by checking the athlete's medical history or medical alert tag.)

The athlete may have suffered a direct blow to the head.

The athlete may be suffering from heatstroke.

The athlete may be suffering from respiratory arrest.

Signs of Minor/Petit Mal Seizures
Dazed or inattentive manner

Confusion

Loss of coordination

Possibly loss of speech

Signs of Major/Grand Mal Seizures (typical sequence)
The body appears stiff or rigid.

Muscles contract violently in spasms or convulsions (see Figure 10.1) that stop generally in 1 to 2 minutes.

The athlete may temporarily stop breathing.

The athlete may lose consciousness.

The breathing is shallow.

There is a bluish appearance to the skin.

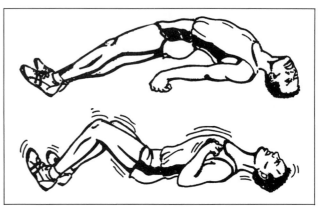

Figure 10.1 Convulsions during a seizure.

First Aid for Minor/Petit Mal Seizures
Monitor the athlete's condition to watch for a major seizure.

Check for signs of other illnesses or injuries.

If there are no other problems and the athlete is a known epileptic, call the parents or guardian to take the athlete home.

First Aid for Major/Grand Mal Seizures
Clear all objects away from the athlete.

Do not try to restrain the athlete or place anything in the athlete's mouth!

After the convulsions stop, check breathing and pulse and provide rescue breathing or CPR if necessary. Check for other possible injuries or illnesses if the athlete is not an epileptic.

If you do not suspect any head or spine injuries, place the athlete on his or her side to allow fluids to drain from the mouth.

Monitor the ABCs and provide rescue breathing or CPR if necessary.

Treat for shock if necessary.

Call the parents or guardian if the athlete is an epileptic and recovers within a few minutes.

If the athlete is suffering from an injury or illness, or does not recover from an epileptic seizure, send for emergency medical assistance.

Encourage the athlete to rest.

Playing Status
Have the athlete rest for the remainder of the day. If the seizure is caused by an injury or illness, the athlete must be released by a physician before returning to activity.

Prevention
Do not allow athletes with acute illnesses to participate until the illness subsides.

Fainting

Definition
Fainting is a temporary loss of consciousness not caused by a head injury.

It can be classified as a mild form of shock.

Cause
It is usually brought on by extreme fatigue, dehydration, low blood pressure, or illness.

History
The athlete suddenly collapses for no apparent reason.

Symptoms
Nausea

Weakness

Headache

Fatigue

Dizziness

Signs
Pale, cool, clammy skin

Possibly shallow and rapid breathing

Possibly loss of consciousness

First Aid for a Conscious Athlete
Have the athlete sit on a chair with his or her head between the knees, as shown in Figure 10.2. Or, have the athlete lie down with the feet elevated.

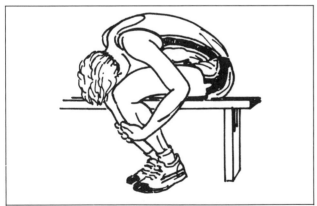

Figure 10.2 Position to prevent fainting.

Treat for shock if necessary.

If the athlete does not recover within a few minutes, send for emergency medical assistance.

First Aid for an Unconscious Athlete
Monitor the ABCs and provide rescue breathing or CPR if necessary.

Send for emergency medical assistance if the athlete does not recover within a few minutes.

Lay the athlete on his or her side to allow fluids to drain from the mouth.

Treat for shock if necessary.

Playing Status
Rest the athlete for the remainder of the day. The athlete must be seen and released by a physician if suffering from an illness.

Prevention
If an athlete feels dizzy, have the athlete sit with the head between the knees, as shown in figure 10.2.

Severe Allergic Reactions (Insect Bites and Stings)

Definition and Cause
Allergies to insect bites or stings can cause sudden illness in some athletes. The severity of the illness depends on how allergic an athlete is to a particular insect. You should be prepared to monitor an athlete and start life-saving first aid if necessary. You may want to review the first aid guidelines for respiratory problems caused by insect bites covered in chapter 7 under "Anaphylactic Shock."

History
The athlete is allergic to certain insects. (You should know this by checking the athlete's medical history or medical alert tag.)

The athlete was stung by an insect.

Symptoms
Itching and/or burning skin around the bite

Weakness

Nausea

Inability to breathe

Abdominal cramps

Possibly chest pain

Dizziness

Signs
Hives

Swelling around the bite

Swelling of the face and tongue (severe reaction)

Labored breathing

Possibly vomiting

Possibly unconsciousness (severe reaction)

Possibly respiratory arrest (severe reaction)

First Aid for a Life-Threatening Allergic Reaction

Use an insect sting kit.

1. Wipe the affected area with an alcohol pad.
2. Give the athlete an epinephrine injection (see kit instructions).
3. Scrape away the stinger with your fingernails or a credit card.
4. If the athlete was stung on the arm or leg, apply the kit's restricting band between the sting and the heart (see kit instructions).
5. Assist the athlete in taking any prescribed antihistamine tablets.
6. Apply ice packs to the sting.
7. Monitor the ABCs and provide rescue breathing or CPR if necessary.
8. Send for emergency medical assistance.
9. Treat for shock if necessary.

First Aid for Mild Allergic Reactions

1. Scrape the stinger away from the skin with your fingernail or a credit card.
2. Apply ice to the sting.
3. Monitor the ABCs and provide rescue breathing or CPR if necessary.
4. Notify the athlete's parents or guardian so they can take the athlete home.

Playing Status

An athlete with a severe reaction cannot return to activity until he or she is released by a physician.

In the case of a minor reaction, the athlete should rest for the remainder of the day.

Prevention

Inspect the playing area for insect nests and spray the area if necessary.

Carry an insect sting emergency kit if one of your athletes has a severe allergy to insect stings.

Encourage athletes with severe allergies to carry their prescribed antihistamine medication.

For Insect Stings

DO NOT ...

. . . squeeze or pinch the area to remove the stinger. This may cause further venom to be released.

Sport First Aid Recap

1. All athletes are prone to sudden illness.

2. Exercise and diet can affect the amount of insulin that the body needs. Thus, diabetic athletes need to be closely monitored for signs of diabetic illness.

3. Insulin shock is caused by a sudden drop in blood sugar levels and therefore requires a quick dose of sugar for first aid.

4. Symptoms and signs of insulin shock include dizziness, headaches, hunger, weakness, pale and cold skin, rapid pulse, confusion, and shock.

5. A diabetic coma is caused by high blood sugar levels and requires prompt assistance by emergency medical personnel.

6. Excessive thirst, dry mouth, headache, abdominal pain, nausea, skin that is red and warm, rapid but weak pulse, and sweet, fruity breath are some of the symptoms and signs of diabetic coma.

7. Alcohol, narcotics, and barbiturates depress the nervous system.

8. An athlete who overdoses on depressants may have cold and clammy skin, a weak and rapid pulse, constricted pupils, and shallow breathing and may possibly suffer from unconsciousness.

9. Cocaine and amphetamines stimulate the nervous system. Athletes on stimulants may be moody, irritable, and confused. They may also have dilated pupils and a rapid pulse, and they may suffer from hallucinations.

10. First aid for either depressant or stimulant overdose consists of sending for medical assistance, monitoring the vital signs, and treating for respiratory or cardiac arrest and shock if necessary.

11. A seizure is an abnormal, excessive electrical discharge from the brain cells.

12. Seizures can be caused by epilepsy, high fever, head injuries, and other conditions.

13. An athlete suffering from a minor/petit mal seizure may appear dazed, confused, and uncoordinated.

14. In major/grand mal seizures, the athlete will suffer convulsions and possibly unconsciousness.

15. Fainting is a temporary loss of consciousness that may be caused by shock, fatigue, dehydration, or illness.

16. Fainting is best prevented and treated by elevating the athlete's feet higher than his or her head.

17. Never take fainting lightly; it may be a sign of a more serious injury or illness.

18. An allergic reaction to a foreign substance such as insect stings may be life-threatening to an athlete. The athlete may develop hives, breathing difficulties, dizziness, chest pain, abdominal cramps, and other signs and symptoms.

19. To minimize the impact of an insect sting, try to clean the area of venom, apply ice to reduce swelling and circulation to the area, and assist the athlete with any allergy medicine that he or she may need.

CHAPTER 11

Temperature-Related Problems

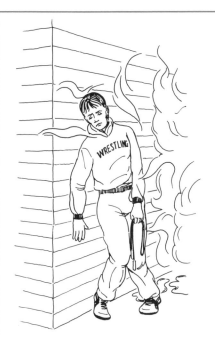

John Gibson is trying to lose two more pounds to qualify for the 138-pound weight class in the next day's regional wrestling tournament. Wearing a vinyl suit, John skips rope in the hot, steamy shower room. He has eaten only soup and drunk very little water today. Just five more minutes on the rope and he is sure the two extra pounds will be history. Then it hits. John begins feeling dizzy and flushed. His head is pounding and his skin feels hot and dry. He stumbles out of the showers in a stupor and collapses on the locker room floor.

No matter where you practice or compete, if the conditions are ripe, one of your athletes could suffer from a heat- or cold-related illness. It may be only 76 degrees and 70% humidity, but an overweight or poorly conditioned athlete could suffer a heat illness. Thin yet highly conditioned athletes may be prone to cold illness because they have less fat to help insulate their bodies. Therefore, it's important for you to be able to recognize, treat, and prevent these conditions.

Before we get into the sport first aid specifics for temperature-related illnesses, let's look at how the body temperature is regulated. Then you will better understand the causes of the specific problems.

Temperature Regulation

There are several different avenues through which the body temperature can rise or fall: metabolism, convection, conduction, radiation, and evaporation. Figure 11.1 gives you a better understanding of what each of these means.

Metabolism

As the tissue cells in the body work and use energy, heat is produced. So, when athletes are active, their body temperatures rise due to an increase in their metabolic rate.

Convection

Convection is the loss or gain of heat resulting from the circulation of air, such as the wind. If the air temperature is warmer than that of the body, the body temperature will increase. If the air temperature is cooler than the body's, then the body temperature will decrease.

Conduction

Body heat can be lost or gained if the body comes in contact with a warmer or colder object. This is the process of conduction. For example, an athlete's body temperature will rise if he or she sits in a warm Jacuzzi. An athlete can lose body heat by coming in contact with a cold shower or by drinking cold water.

Radiation

Radiation is heat lost or gained through contact with infrared waves. The most common form of radiation heat is from the sun. The degree of cloudiness and the angle of the sun are just two of the variables that can determine the radiative effects of the sun.

Evaporation

Active athletes as well as those in hot or humid conditions typically perspire a great deal. Evaporation of sweat off the skin is the main way in which the body cools itself.

Heat-Related Illnesses

How many road races are run after 11 a.m.? Not many, especially during the summer months and in warm, humid weather. Experience tells us that even highly fit athletes succumb to sweltering conditions. Here's why.

On hot, humid days the body has difficulty cooling itself. Because the air is already saturated with water vapor (humidity), sweat doesn't evaporate as easily. Therefore, the body sweat is a less effective cooling agent, and the body retains extra heat. It is this combination of increased metabolism and decreased evaporation of sweat that makes

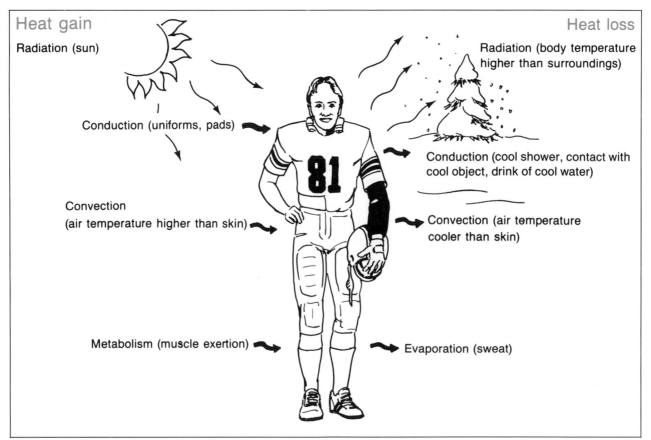

Figure 11.1 Means of heat gain and loss.

athletes more prone to heat illness in hot, humid environments. In addition, athletes often wear heavy equipment or pads that also hinder the evaporation of sweat, making them even more susceptible to heat-related problems.

THREE TYPES OF HEAT ILLNESS

- Heat cramps
- Heat exhaustion
- Heatstroke

Prevention of Heat-Related Illnesses

Obviously, the weather conditions are not always going to be ideal for every practice and competition. So if you are located in a warm-weather climate or have practices during the summer, you'll have to take preventive measures.

- *Monitor weather conditions and adjust practices accordingly.*
  Figure 11.2 shows the specific air temperatures and humidity percentages that can be hazardous. It also provides guidelines for modifying your practices to reduce the risk of heat illness.

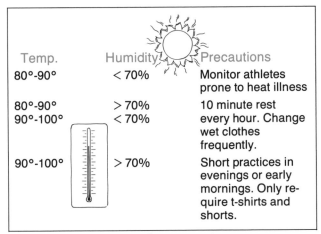

Temp.	Humidity	Precautions
80°-90°	< 70%	Monitor athletes prone to heat illness
80°-90°	> 70%	10 minute rest every hour. Change wet clothes frequently.
90°-100°	< 70%	
90°-100°	> 70%	Short practices in evenings or early mornings. Only require t-shirts and shorts.

Figure 11.2 Warm-weather precautions.

- *Acclimatize athletes to exercising in high heat and humidity.*
  Athletes will adjust to high heat and humidity if given time, approximately 7 to 10 days. During this time, hold short practices at low to moderate activity levels and give the athletes water breaks every 20 minutes.
- *Switch to light clothing and less equipment.*
  Athletes will stay cooler if they wear shorts, white T-shirts, and less equipment. Equipment makes it hard for sweat to evaporate. Absolutely forbid athletes to wear vinyl sweatsuits at any time! Vinyl prevents evaporation of sweat and therefore does not allow the body to cool itself. This practice is especially popular with wrestlers and boxers.
- *Identify and monitor athletes who are prone to heat illness.*
  Athletes who are overweight, heavily muscled, or out of shape are prone to heat illness. Athletes who have suffered from a previous heat illness or who work out extremely hard are also at risk. These athletes should be closely monitored and given water breaks every 15 to 20 minutes.
- *Make sure athletes replace body fluids (water) lost through sweat.*
  Athletes can lose a great deal of water through sweat. If this fluid is not replaced, the body will have less water to cool itself with (dehydration). Don't rely on athletes to drink enough fluids on their own. They won't actually feel thirsty until they've lost 3% to 4% of their body weight in sweat (water). However, athletic performance may worsen after only 2% of the body weight is lost through sweat. Therefore, encourage athletes to do the following:

  Drink 1 liter of water each day.

  Drink 8 ounces (or 1 cup) of water every 15 minutes during practice or competition.

  Drink 1/2 to 1 cup of water 15 minutes before practice or competition.

  Also encourage athletes to weigh themselves before and after practice or competition. They should drink 2 cups of water for every pound of water they've lost through sweat.

  Cool water is the best fluid to drink because the stomach absorbs it faster than it does electrolyte (sport) drinks.
- *Replenish electrolytes lost through sweat.*
  Electrolytes such as sodium (salt) and potassium are also lost through sweat. These are used in muscle contraction and

other body functions, and they must be replaced. The best way for athletes to replace these nutrients is by eating a normal diet that contains fresh fruits and vegetables. Bananas are a good source of potassium. Athletes can replace sodium by lightly salting their food. The typical American diet contains more salt than the body needs, so athletes don't have to go overboard with the salt shaker.

Identifying and Treating Heat-Related Illnesses

Each of the different forms of heat illness have different signs and symptoms, as well as different first aid interventions. Heatstroke is life-threatening, whereas heat exhaustion and heat cramps typically are not. Therefore, it is important that you learn to evaluate and apply the first aid techniques that are appropriate for each illness.

Heat Cramps

Definition
This condition involves sudden involuntary muscle spasms.

Causes
Dehydration

Electrolyte loss

Poor or decreased blood flow to the muscles

History
The athlete complains of a muscle spasm that is not caused by a specific injury.

Cramps usually occur in the quadriceps, hamstrings, or calves.

Symptoms
Pain caused by muscle spasm

Fatigue

Signs
Severe muscle spasms

First Aid
Have the athlete rest.

Instruct the athlete to slowly stretch the affected muscle without bouncing. See Appendix B for correct stretching techniques.

Have the athlete drink cool water.

If the spasms do not improve within 5 minutes, look for another possible injury, and send the athlete to a physician.

Playing Status
The athlete can return to activity once the spasms stop and he or she can run, jump, and cut without limping or pain.

Heat Exhaustion

Definition
This is a shocklike condition.

Cause
Dehydration occurs when the body's water and electrolyte supplies are depleted through sweating.

History
The athlete suffered no injury but begins to develop shocklike symptoms.

Symptoms
Headache

Nausea

Dizziness

Chills

Fatigue

Extreme thirst

Signs
Pale, cool, and clammy skin

Rapid, weak pulse

Loss of coordination

Dilated pupils

Profuse sweating (key sign)

First Aid
Have the athlete rest in a cool, shaded area.

Give the athlete cool water to drink (if he or she is conscious).

You can apply ice to the athlete's neck, back, or stomach to help cool the body.

Monitor the athlete's ABCs and provide rescue breathing or CPR if necessary.

Treat for shock if necessary.

Send for emergency medical assistance if the athlete does not recover or if his or her condition worsens.

If the athlete recovers, call the parents or guardian to take the athlete home.

Playing Status
The athlete cannot return to activity until she or he regains the weight lost through sweat. This may take several days. An athlete absolutely must not return to activity on the same day that he or she suffered heat exhaustion. If the athlete is sent to a physician or does not quickly recover, do not allow him or her to return to activity until released by a physician.

Heatstroke

Definition
This is a life-threatening condition in which the body stops sweating and the body temperature rises dangerously high.

Cause
Dehydration causes a malfunction in the body's temperature control center in the brain.

History
The athlete may dazedly stagger off the field or collapse.

Symptoms
Feeling of being on fire (extremely hot)

Nausea

Confusion

Irritability

Fatigue

Signs
Hot, dry, and flushed or red skin (key sign)

Very high body temperature (above 103 degrees)

Lack of sweat

Rapid pulse

Rapid breathing

Constricted pupils

Vomiting

Diarrhea

Possibly seizures

Possibly unconsciousness

Possibly respiratory or cardiac arrest

First Aid
Send for emergency medical assistance.

Have the athlete rest in a cool, shaded area.

Remove excess clothing and equipment.

Cool the athlete's body with cool, wet towels or by pouring cool water over him or her.

Apply ice packs to the athlete's armpits, neck, back, stomach, and between the legs.

Monitor the ABCs and provide rescue breathing or CPR if necessary.

Treat for shock if necessary (**do not** cover the athlete with blankets).

Have a conscious athlete drink cool water.

Place an unconscious or incoherent athlete on his or her side to allow fluids and vomit to drain from the mouth.

Playing Status
The athlete cannot return to activity until he or she is released by a physician.

Because heatstroke is a life-threatening condition, it's important for you to recognize the signs and symptoms highlighted in Figure 11.3 and to be prepared to provide immediate first aid care. The illustration will also help you review the basic differences between heat exhaustion and heatstroke.

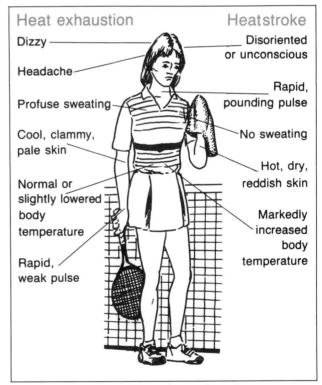

Figure 11.3 Heatstroke vs. heat exhaustion.

Cold-Related Illnesses

Bud Grant, former coach of the National Football League's Minnesota Vikings, used to forbid portable heaters on the sidelines, even on the coldest days in Bloomington, Minnesota. Those afternoons were true tests of both the players' and fans' ability to survive under freezing conditions. But more than a few victims suffered frostbite on those Sunday afternoons. So now, perhaps not surprisingly, the Vikings play all of their home games indoors.

When a person is exposed to cold weather, like that which Minnesota experiences in the falls and winters, the body temperature starts to drop below normal. To counteract this, the body tries to gain or conserve heat by shivering and reducing the blood flow. Shivering involves muscles contracting rapidly to produce heat. At the same time, the reduction of blood flow to the skin and extremities conserves the heat of the brain, heart, and lungs.

Prevention of Cold-Related Illnesses

But no matter how effective the body's natural heating mechanism is, the body will better withstand cold temperatures if it is prepared to handle them. Following are some precautions that you and your players can take to reduce your risk of cold-related illnesses.

- *Make sure athletes wear appropriate protective clothing.*
  Athletes should dress in layers, which allows sweat to evaporate and protects against the cold. Wool, Gortex, and Lycra are excellent materials to wear. Also, be sure the head and neck are covered to prevent excessive heat loss.

  Mittens are preferable to gloves because they allow the fingers to warm each other.
- *Keep athletes active to maintain body heat.*
  Athletes who must stand along the sidelines should keep moving to help produce body heat. Jumping up and down and jogging in place are good sideline exercises.
- *Monitor the windchill* (see Figure 11.4).

TWO COMMON COLD-RELATED ILLNESSES

- Frostbite
- Hypothermia

		Temperature (°F)								
		0	5	10	15	20	25	30	35	40
Wind speed (mph)		Flesh may freeze within 1 minute								
	40	-55	-45	-35	-30	-20	-15	-5	0	10
	35	-50	-40	-35	-30	-20	-10	-5	5	10
	30	-50	-40	-30	-25	-20	-10	0	5	10
	25	-45	-35	-30	-20	-15	-5	0	10	15
	20	-35	-30	-25	-15	-10	0	5	10	20
	15	-30	-25	-20	-10	-5	0	10	15	25
	10	-20	-15	-10	0	5	10	15	20	30
	5	-5	0	5	10	15	20	25	30	35
		Windchill temperature (°F)								

Figure 11.4 Windchill factor index.

Identifying and Treating Cold-Related Illnesses

Frostbite and hypothermia each have specific signs and symptoms that you need to know. The first aid that you administer will depend on which condition the athlete has and will dictate how well the athlete recovers from the condition.

Frostbite

Definition
Superficial frostbite involves localized freezing of the skin and the superficial tissues below it. The nose, ears, toes, and fingers are especially prone to superficial frostbite. Deep frostbite begins superficially but advances to deep tissues such as muscles and tendons.

Cause
Exposure of body parts to cold, causing tissues to freeze and blood vessels to constrict

Symptoms
Painful, itchy, burning, or tingling areas that may become numb as the frostbite worsens. These symptoms may recur when the affected areas are rewarmed.

Signs

First-degree frostbite—red or flushed skin that may turn white or gray

Second-degree frostbite—firm, white, and waxy skin
Blisters and purple tint to skin may appear when the area is rewarmed.

Third-degree frostbite—blisters
Bluish skin
The area feels very cold and stiff.

First Aid
Move the athlete to a warm area.

Remove wet and cold clothing.

Treat for shock if necessary.

First- and Second-Degree Frostbite
Rewarm frostbitten areas by soaking them in clean, warm water (100 to 105 degrees).

Call the athlete's parents or guardian to take the athlete to a physician.

Third-Degree Frostbite
Send for emergency medical assistance.

Monitor the ABCs and provide rescue breathing or CPR if necessary.

Cover the frostbitten areas with sterile gauze.

Playing Status
The athlete cannot return to activity until he or she is released by a physician.

For Frostbite

DO NOT . . .
. . . rub or massage frostbitten areas.
. . . apply ice to frostbitten areas.
. . . allow frostbitten tissue to refreeze.

Hypothermia

Definition
In this condition, the body temperature drops below normal.

Causes
Prolonged exposure to wet, windy, and cold environment

Extreme fatigue, such as that suffered after competition in a marathon or triathlon

History
The athlete did not suffer an injury but begins to act irrational and disoriented.

Symptoms
When the body temperature drops below 95 degrees:

Irritability

Confusion

Drowsiness

Lethargy

Signs

From 95 degrees to 98.6 degrees:
Loss of coordination
Loss of sensation
Uncontrollable shivering

From 90 to 95 degrees:
Shivering may stop
Pale and hard skin
Numbness
Slow, irregular pulse
Slowed breathing

From 86 to 90 degrees:
  Hallucinations
  Dilated pupils
Below 85 degrees:
  Unconsciousness
  Respiratory arrest

First Aid

Mild to Moderate Hypothermia
  Move the athlete to a warm area.
  Send for emergency medical assistance.
  Gently remove cold and wet clothes.
  Wrap the athlete in blankets.
  Give warm fluids, such as hot tea or cider,
    to a conscious athlete.

Severe Hypothermia
  Send for emergency medical assistance.
  Cover the athlete with blankets.
  Treat the athlete very carefully. Excessive
    movements or jarring may cause cold
    blood to recirculate to the heart. This
    can cause the heart to stop.
  Monitor the ABCs and provide rescue
    breathing or CPR if necessary.
  Treat for shock.

Playing Status
The athlete cannot return to activity until he
or she is released by a physician.

Sport First Aid Recap

1. Heat- and cold-related illness can have a negative affect on your athletes' health as well as their performance.

2. The body gains or loses heat through metabolism, convection, conduction, radiation, and evaporation.

3. Three common types of heat illness are heat cramps, heat exhaustion, and heatstroke.

4. Heat exhaustion is a serious heat illness that can cause shock-like signs and symptoms.

5. Heatstroke is a life-threatening illness that shuts down the body's sweating mechanism, causing the body temperature to rise to dangerously high levels.

6. Preventive measures such as adjusting practice locations and times to weather conditions, acclimatizing athletes to high heat and humidity, instructing athletes to wear light clothing, monitoring athletes at risk, and having athletes replenish the body's water supplies will help reduce the incidence of heat illness.

7. You can prevent cold-related illnesses by making sure athletes wear layers of warm clothing and stay active, and by monitoring the windchill.

8. Frostbite is a superficial (skin and subskin tissue) or deep (muscle and other deep tissue) freezing of body tissues.

9. Treatment for frostbite involves moving the athlete to a warmer environment and slowly rewarming the frostbitten areas in warm water.

10. Hypothermia is a life-threatening condition in which the body temperature drops below normal.

11. First aid for hypothermia includes rewarming the body, monitoring breathing and pulse rates, and treating for shock.

12. Any athlete who has a previous history of either a cold- or a heat-related illness is particularly prone to suffering the same condition again.

CHAPTER 12

Musculoskeletal Injuries

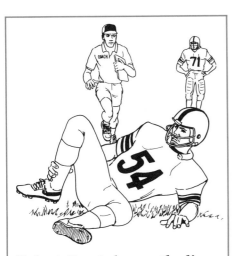

Robert Grant charges the line of scrimmage to grasp the ball carrier. Just as he moves in for the tackle, however, the elusive runner cuts to the outside. Robert has to pivot quickly to make the stop. But as he lunges for the opponent, the cleats on his right shoe catch on the ground, forcing his ankle to roll over. Robert's coach, Ron Town, is faced with evaluating and administering first aid to Robert's injured ankle. What should he do?

The majority of athletic sport injuries are musculoskeletal in nature—things like sprains, strains, fractures, dislocations, and tendinitis. Because of their prevalence, you should be especially prepared to administer to muscle- and bone-related problems. Perhaps it will help to refer back to chapter 3 and review these types of injuries before you proceed. Then, when you are comfortable with your knowledge of that material, progress through this chapter and learn how to evaluate and apply first aid to the many types of musculoskeletal injuries that can occur.

Musculoskeletal Injury Plan

Regardless of the type of musculoskeletal injury that an athlete suffers, the evaluation you make and the first aid you apply will be much the same in all cases. Therefore, let's first establish some general procedures for evaluating and handling these injuries.

Evaluation Guidelines

It's best to sort out injuries according to their severity and nature of development. To help you do this, in Table 12.1 musculoskeletal injuries are classified into three levels of severity: acute mild, acute Grade II and III, and chronic. In addition, we've listed evaluation findings and first aid guidelines for each category. Keep in mind that these are *general* directives, but notice the difference in the signs, symptoms, and first aid for each injury level.

Remember, chronic injuries (tendinitis, bursitis, and some Grade I strains) develop gradually, whereas acute injuries (sprains and Grade II and III strains) develop suddenly. Consequently, pain, swelling, and loss of function

Table 12.1   General Guidelines for Musculoskeletal Injuries

	Acute mild (sprains, strains, contusions)	Grade II and III (sprains, strains, contusions, fractures, dislocations)	Chronic (bursitis, tendinitis, stress fractures)
Common evaluation findings			
Mechanism			
Sudden	X	X	
Gradual			X
Signs			
Swelling	X	X	May be delayed
Deformity	Not likely	X	Not likely
Discoloration	X	X	Not likely
Warm to touch		Possible	X
Muscle spasm	Very mild	Severe	Mild to moderate
Tenderness to touch	X	Extreme point	Diffuse tenderness
Loss of motion	Slight	X	Delayed
Symptoms			
Pain	X	X	X
Grating		X	X
Numbness	X	X	X
Popping	X	X	X
First aid			
PRICE	X	X	X
Immobilization		X	If stress fracture
Monitor heart/breathing		X	
Treat shock	X	X	
Medical attention	If signs and symptoms persist	X	If signs and symptoms persist

X indicates that the evaluation or first aid applies to the problem.

will occur suddenly in acute injuries and more slowly—over a period of days or weeks—in chronic injuries. Also, chronic injuries are not caused by a specific injury but develop from overuse, muscle weakness, and inflexibility.

First Aid Guidelines

Suppose Robert Grant—the would-be tackler in the chapter-opening scenario, had a moderately swollen ankle. The injury also resulted in slight point tenderness and loss of function. It's probably a Grade II ankle sprain, right? Not necessarily.

The signs and symptoms of Grade II and III ligament sprains, Grade III muscle strains, severe contusions, and dislocations are similar to those of a fracture. Therefore, the safest approach is to always assume that an injury of this nature is a fracture, and treat it as such.

It is very difficult to differentiate between a fracture and any of these other injuries; they all can result in swelling, pain, deformity, discoloration, and loss of motion. Sometimes, fractures will distinguish themselves by their gross deformity and grating sensations. But for your purposes, it's not important to determine exactly whether an injury is a sprain, strain, fracture, contusion, or dislocation. What **is** important is that you treat all such injuries with PRICE (see p. 59) and immobilization, then see to it that they are examined by a physician. The general guidelines recommended in Table 12.1 will help you handle your athletes' common musculoskeletal injuries in an appropriate manner.

Now that you know how to classify and treat musculoskeletal injuries in general, let's look at how you should address specific injuries. The remainder of this chapter is divided by body parts, with complete sport first aid guidelines for the acute and chronic musculoskeletal problems that may afflict athletes at each site. Beginning at the shoulder, we'll proceed down to the feet, looking at the most common sport injuries along the way.

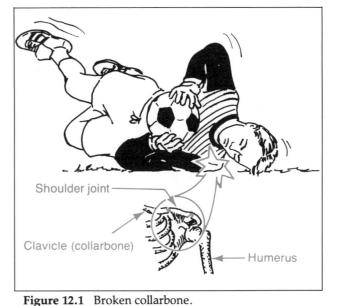

Figure 12.1 Broken collarbone.

Shoulder

Acute shoulder injuries commonly occur in football and wrestling, whereas chronic shoulder injuries typically occur in volleyball, swimming, baseball, and softball. In wrestling, for example, shoulder injuries are the number-one type of injury among high school wrestlers (NATA, 1989b) and account for 10.3% of all injuries sustained by high school football players (NATA, 1989a). Because of their high rate of occurrence in sport, and especially in contact sports, it's important that you are able to evaluate and provide first aid for shoulder injuries.

Acute Shoulder Injuries

Broken Collarbone (Clavicle)

Cause
Direct blow to the front or side of the shoulder

Symptom
Pain in the front of the shoulder along the collarbone

Sign
Deformity of the collarbone (see Figure 12.1)

First Aid
Send for medical assistance.

Immobilize the arm with a sling.

Secure the arm to the body with an elastic wrap.

Treat for shock if necessary.

Gently apply ice over the area for 15 minutes.

Playing Status
The athlete cannot return to activity until he or she is released by a physician and has full shoulder strength, motion, and flexibility.

Prevention
Require athletes to wear shoulder pads if they are part of the standard equipment.

Have athletes avoid direct blows to the side of the shoulder.

A/C Sprain (Shoulder Separation)

Definition
This is a stretch or tear of the ligaments that connect the collarbone to the shoulder blade (see Figure 12.2).

Cause
Direct blow to the top of the shoulder, similar to that illustrated in Figure 12.2

Symptom
Pain along the outer edge of the collarbone

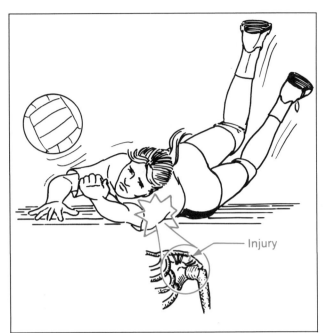

Figure 12.2 Acromioclavicular (A/C) sprain.

Sign
Deformity along the outer edge of the collarbone

First Aid
Send for medical assistance.

Immobilize the arm with a sling.

Secure the arm to the body with an elastic wrap.

Treat for shock if necessary.

Gently apply ice over the area for 15 minutes.

Playing Status
The athlete cannot return to activity until he or she is released by a physician and has full shoulder strength, motion, and flexibility.

The athlete should wear a special protective pad over the injury once he or she returns to activity.

Shoulder Dislocation or Subluxation

Definition
In a dislocation, the upper arm bone (humerus) moves out of the shoulder joint socket located on the shoulder blade (scapula) as shown in Figure 12.3.

In a subluxation, the same thing occurs, except the humerus immediately goes back into the socket.

Cause
Direct upward blow to the shoulder

Backward blow to the shoulder while the upper arm is flexed forward, as shown in Figure 12.3.

Forceful contraction of the shoulder muscles.

Symptom
Intense pain where the upper arm bone connects to the shoulder blade

Signs
Possibly numbness in the arm caused by the displaced bone pinching nerves and arteries

Inability to move the arm

Shoulder appears flat instead of rounded

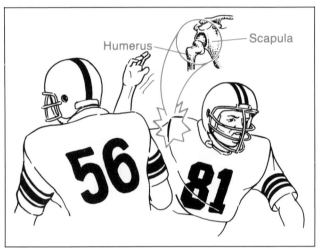

Figure 12.3 Shoulder dislocation.

First Aid
Send for medical assistance.

Stabilize the arm in the position in which you found it.

Do not try to put the upper arm bone back into the socket.

Treat for shock as necessary.

Gently apply ice over the area for 15 minutes.

Playing Status
The athlete cannot participate until he or she is released by a physician; the shoulder is pain-free; and he or she has normal motion, strength, and flexibility.

S/C Sprain (Shoulder Separation)

Definition
This is a stretch or tear of the ligaments that

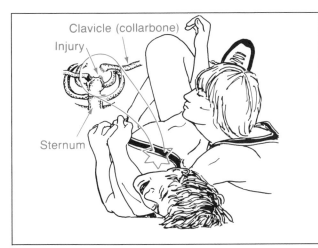

Figure 12.4 Sternoclavicular (S/C) sprain.

connect the collarbone to the breastbone (see Figure 12.4).

Causes
Falling on an outstretched hand

Direct blow that pushes the shoulder forward

Symptom
Major blood vessels and nerves to the brain run behind this joint through the neck. If the injury is severe, check for dizziness.

Signs
Tenderness at the attachment of the collarbone to the breastbone

Deformity at the attachment of the collarbone to the breastbone

Severe sprain may cause nerve and artery damage

Possibly unconsciousness

Respiratory or cardiac arrest

First Aid
Send for emergency medical assistance.

Monitor the athlete's ABCs and provide rescue breathing and CPR if necessary.

Treat for shock if necessary.

Immobilize the arm with a sling.

Secure the arm to the body with an elastic wrap.

Gently apply ice over the area for 15 minutes.

Playing Status
The athlete cannot return to activity until he or she is released by a physician and has normal shoulder strength, motion, and flexibility.

The athlete should wear a protective pad over the injury when he or she returns to activity.

Chronic Shoulder Injuries

Rotator Cuff Strain

Definition
This is a stretch or tear of the rotator cuff muscles used in throwing (see Figure 12.5).

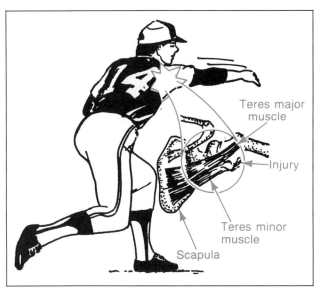

Figure 12.5 Rotator cuff strain.

Cause
Chronic overuse of the rotator cuff. This can happen if an athlete throws hard or incorrectly with weak and inflexible shoulder muscles.

Symptom
Pain with throwing, spiking, and serving motions

Signs
Inability to throw, spike, or serve with a normal throwing pattern

Tenderness over the front of the shoulder, just below the edge of the collarbone, or along the shoulder blade

First Aid
Have the athlete rest until seen by a physician.

Gently apply ice over the area for 15 minutes.

Playing Status
The athlete cannot return to activity until he

or she is released by a physician and has full shoulder strength, motion, and flexibility.

Prevention
Have the athlete undergo preseason strengthening and stretching of the shoulder.

Have the athlete gradually begin throwing, starting with slow speed and short distance throws, and gradually increasing the speed and distance. This should take 1 to 2 weeks.

Impingement Syndrome

Definition
The tendons of the rotator cuff become swollen and get pinched underneath the collarbone.

Cause
Overuse of weak or inflexible shoulder muscles. The tendons become swollen and are pinched by the collarbone when the arm is raised.

Symptoms
Pain when the arm is raised overhead (key symptom)

Aching pain during and/or after activity

Tenderness just below the outer edge of the collarbone on the front of the shoulder

First Aid
Have the athlete rest until seen by a physician.

Gently apply ice over the area for 15 minutes.

Playing Status
The athlete cannot return to activity until he or she is released by a physician and has normal shoulder strength, motion, and flexibility.

Prevention
Have the athlete undergo preseason strengthening and flexibility training for the shoulder.

Have the athlete start throwing, serving, spiking, or swimming for short distances and at slow speeds, and gradually increase the distance and speed.

Shoulder Injury Summary

The six injuries just presented are the most common shoulder injuries in sport. For your convenience, Table 12.2 summarizes the evaluation and care for athletes who suffer these acute and chronic shoulder problems.

Elbow

The elbow is most often injured in tennis, baseball, softball, and wrestling. Tennis, baseball, and softball players are most susceptible to chronic injuries such as tennis elbow, whereas wrestlers are more prone to acute injuries such as a dislocation. The next few pages will introduce you to the most common acute and chronic injuries and inform you of how to provide emergency care for them.

Acute Elbow Injuries

Elbow Fracture

Definition
This is a break of any or all of the bones that make up the elbow. This includes the upper

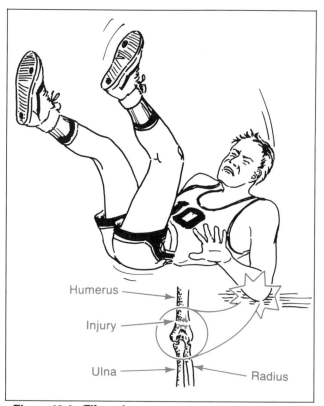

Figure 12.6 Elbow fracture.

Table 12.2   First Aid Summary for Shoulder Injuries

	Acute				Chronic	
	Clavicle fracture	A/C separation	Shoulder dislocation	S/C separation	Rotator cuff strain	Impingement
Common evaluation findings						
Mechanism						
Sudden	X	X	X	X	X	
Gradual					X	X
Signs						
Swelling	X	X	X	X		
Deformity	X	X	X	X		
Discoloration						
Warm to touch						
Muscle spasm	X	X	X	X		
Tenderness to touch	X	X	X	X	X	X
Loss of motion	X	X	X	X	X	X
Symptoms						
Pain	X	X	X	X	X	X
Grating	X	X	Possible	X		
Numbness	X		X			
Popping		X	X	Possible	Possible	Possible
First aid						
PRICE	X	X	X	X	X	X
Immobilization	X	X	X	X		
Monitor ABCs	X	X	X	X		
Treat shock	X	X	X	X		
Medical attention	X	X	X	X	X	X

X indicates that the evaluation or first aid applies to the problem.

arm bone (humerus; see Figure 12.6) and two forearm bones (radius and ulna).

Cause
Direct blow to the area

Symptoms
Possibly numbness and coldness around the area and in the forearm and hand

Signs
Tenderness over the elbow bones

Possibly a deformity at the elbow

First Aid
Send for emergency medical assistance.

Stabilize the arm in the position in which you found it.

Secure the arm to the body with an elastic wrap.

Treat for shock if necessary.

Gently apply ice over the area for 15 minutes.

Playing Status
The athlete cannot return to activity until he or she is released by a physician and has normal elbow strength, motion, and flexibility.

Prevention
Make sure athletes wear protective elbow pads.

Elbow Contusion

Definition
The soft tissues or bones of the elbow joint are bruised.

This is sometimes called "hitting the funny bone."

Cause
Direct blow to the elbow

Symptom
Possibly numbness or tingling down the forearm and hand (a nerve is bruised)

Signs
Possibly swelling or discoloration at the contused area

Tenderness over the contusion

First Aid
Immobilize the arm in the position in which you found it if pain and loss of motion are moderate to severe.

Send for emergency medical assistance if necessary.

Treat for shock if necessary.

Gently apply ice over the area for 15 minutes.

Playing Status
For moderate to severe contusions, the athlete cannot return to activity until he or she is released by a physician and has normal elbow strength, motion, and flexibility.

Prevention
Make sure athletes wear protective elbow pads in football, hockey, basketball, and volleyball.

Elbow Sprain

Definition
This is a stretch or tear of the ligament(s) holding the elbow bones together (see Figure 12.7).

Cause
Direct blow or twisting injury that forces the elbow sideways or backward

Symptom
Possibly numbness or tingling down the forearm and hand (a nerve is injured)

Signs
Tenderness over the sides and back of the elbow

Possibly swelling in moderate and severe cases

First Aid
For Grade II and III sprains, immobilize the elbow in the position in which you found it.

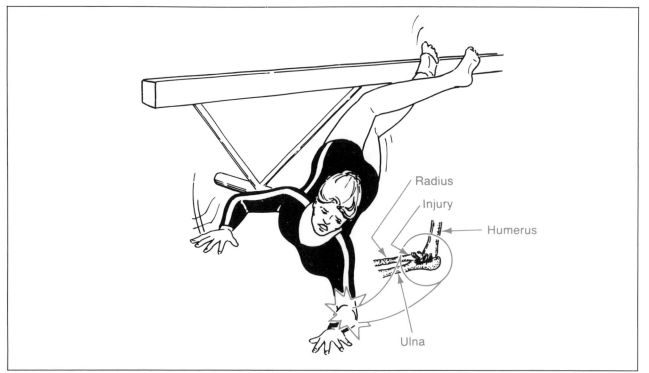

Figure 12.7 Elbow sprain.

Send for emergency medical assistance if pain and loss of motion are moderate to severe.

Treat for shock if necessary.

Gently apply ice over the area for 15 minutes.

Playing Status
For Grade II and III sprains, the athlete cannot return to activity until he or she is released by a physician and has normal elbow strength, motion, and flexibility.

Prevention
Have athletes undergo preseason strengthening and flexibility training.

Elbow Dislocation or Subluxation

Definition
The bone(s) of the elbow joint move out of place and either remain out of place (dislocation) or move back into normal position (subluxation).

Causes
Direct blow to the elbow

Falling on an outstretched hand

Severe elbow sprain

Symptom
Possibly numbness or tingling down the forearm and hand (a nerve is pinched)

Signs
Extreme tenderness around the elbow

Possibly elbow in a slightly bent position

Possibly swelling or other deformity around the elbow area

First Aid
Send for emergency medical assistance.

Immobilize the elbow in the position in which you found it.

Treat for shock if necessary.

Gently apply ice over the area for 15 minutes.

Playing Status
The athlete cannot return to activity until he or she is released by a physician and has normal strength, motion, and flexibility.

The athlete may need protective taping or bracing for the elbow once he or she returns to activity.

Prevention
Have athletes undergo preseason strengthening and flexibility training.

Chronic Elbow Injuries

Tennis Elbow

Definition
This is a chronic strain and/or inflammation where the wrist muscles attach on the outside of the elbow joint (see Figure 12.8).

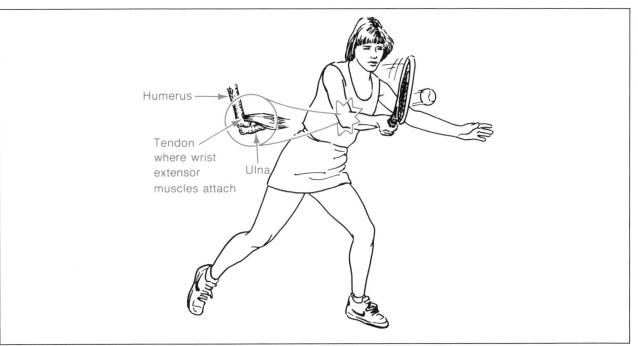

Figure 12.8   Tennis elbow.

Cause
Overuse of weak or inflexible wrist muscles. The muscles and tendons may also be gradually stretched or torn.

Symptom
Pain typically with backhand strokes in racquetball and tennis

Signs
Possibly an inability to lift objects with the injured arm

Possibly swelling over the outside of the elbow

Point tenderness over the outside of the elbow

First Aid
Have the athlete rest the elbow until he or she is seen and released by a physician.

For moderate to severe pain and loss of function, immobilize the elbow with an arm sling.

Gently apply ice over the area for 15 minutes.

Playing Status
For moderate to severe cases, the athlete cannot return to activity until he or she is released by a physician and has normal strength, motion, and flexibility.

Prevention
Have athletes undergo preseason strengthening and flexibility training.

Elbow Growth Plate Stress Fracture

Definition
There is a break in the growth plate of the upper arm bone (humerus) at the elbow (see Figure 12.9).

Cause
Overuse by repetitive and forceful throwing weakens the growth plate until it breaks.

Symptom
Pain gradually worsens over the inside edge of the elbow.

Signs
Possibly swelling or a deformity over the elbow

Point tenderness over the inside of the elbow

First Aid
If pain and loss of function are moderate to severe, immobilize the elbow in a nonpainful position.

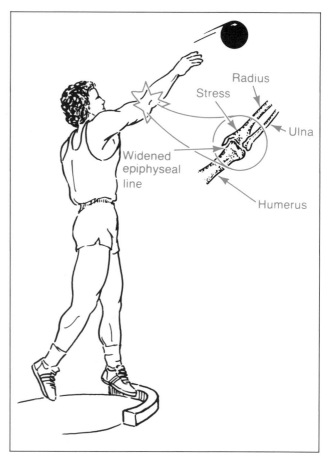

Figure 12.9 Elbow growth plate fracture.

Treat for shock if necessary.

Gently apply ice over the area for 15 minutes.

Playing Status
Have the athlete rest the elbow until he or she is seen and released by a physician.

Prevention
Have athletes undergo preseason strengthening and flexibility training.

Limit forceful throwing by growing athletes.

Elbow Bursitis

Definition
This is an inflammation of the elbow bursa, as shown in Figure 12.10.

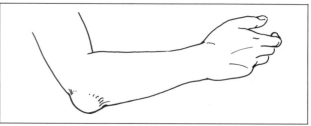

Figure 12.10 Elbow bursitis.

Causes
Single or repetitive blows to the elbow

Infection

Symptom
Pain along the back of the elbow

Signs
Gradual or sudden swelling on the back of the elbow

Noticeable bump on the back of the elbow

Bump may feel warm

First Aid
Rest.

Have the athlete rest the elbow until he or she is seen and released by a physician.

Gently apply ice over the area for 15 minutes.

Playing Status
The athlete cannot return to activity until he or she is released by a physician and has normal strength, motion, and flexibility.

The athlete should wear a protective elbow pad once he or she returns to activity.

Prevention
Require athletes who are prone to hitting their elbows to wear elbow pads.

Elbow Injury Summary

The acute and chronic elbow injuries that we've covered in this section may prevent athletes from participating, particularly in throwing, swinging, and lifting sports. Use Table 12.3 to help you evaluate and administer first aid for each of these elbow injuries.

Forearm, Wrist, and Hand

Almost all of the sport injuries involving the forearm, wrist, and hand are acute. Volleyball, basketball, baseball, softball, and football players are especially prone to such injuries. Following are the most common acute forearm, wrist, and hand problems in sport.

Forearm Fracture

Definition
This is a break in one or both forearm bones, as shown in Figure 12.11.

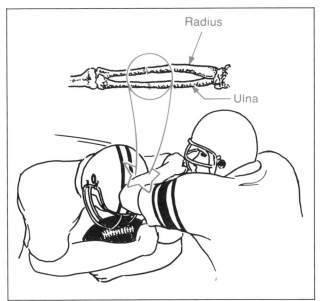

Figure 12.11   Forearm fracture.

Causes
Direct blow to the forearm

Falling on an outstretched hand

Symptom
Pain around the forearm

Signs
Swelling and possibly deformity

Tenderness over the injured area

First Aid
Send for emergency medical assistance.

Splint the arm in the position in which you found it.

Treat for shock if necessary.

Gently apply ice over the area for 15 minutes.

Playing Status
The athlete cannot return to activity until he or she is released by a physician and has normal arm strength, motion, and flexibility.

Prevention
Make sure athletes wear protective forearm pads in football and hockey.

Wrist Sprain

Definition
This is a stretch or tear of the ligament(s) that hold the wrist bones together (see Figure 12.12).

Causes
Twisting injury of the wrist

Table 12.3   First Aid Summary for Elbow Injuries

	Acute				Chronic		
	Fracture	Contusion	Sprain	Dislocation/ subluxation	Tennis elbow	Stress fracture	Bursitis
Common evaluation findings							
Mechanism							
Sudden	X	X	X	X			X
Gradual					X	X	X
Signs							
Swelling	X	X	X	X	Possible	X	X
Deformity	X			X		Possible	
Discoloration	X	X	Possible	X		Possible	
Warm to touch							X
Muscle spasm	X	X	X	X		Possible	
Tenderness to touch	X	X	X	X	X	X	X
Loss of motion	X	Possible	X	X	Possible	X	X
Symptoms							
Pain	X	X	X	X	X	X	X
Grating	X			X		Possible	X
Numbness	X	X	X	X	X		
Popping	X		Possible	X		Possible	Possible
First aid							
PRICE	X	X	X	X	X	X	X
Immobilization	X	If severe	G. II & III	X	If severe	X	
Monitor heart/breathing	X		G. II & III	X		X	
Treat shock	X		G. II & III	X		X	
Medical attention	X	If severe	X	X	X	X	X

X indicates that the evaluation or first aid applies to the problem.

G. = Grade

Falling on an outstretched hand

Signs
Generalized pain around the wrist

Possibly swelling

First Aid
For Grade II and III sprains, have the athlete rest until seen and released by a physician.

If pain and loss of motion are severe, immobilize the wrist.

Secure the arm to the body with an arm sling.

Treat for shock if necessary.

Gently apply ice over the area for 15 minutes.

Playing Status
For Grade II and III sprains, the athlete cannot return to activity until he or she is released by a physician and has normal wrist strength, motion, and flexibility.

The athlete may use protective taping for the wrist when he or she returns to activity.

If pain continues with activity, the athlete should be reevaluated for a possible navicular (small wrist bone) fracture.

Prevention
Have athletes undergo preseason strength and flexibility training.

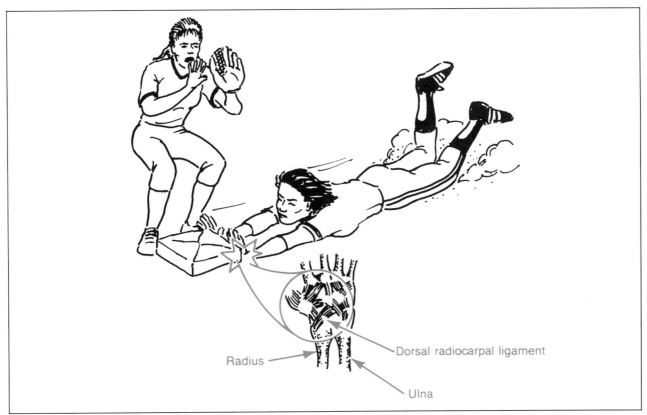

Radius

Dorsal radiocarpal ligament

Ulna

Figure 12.12 Wrist sprain.

Hand Fracture

Definition
There is a break in the bone(s) of the hand, such as that illustrated in Figure 12.13.

Causes
Direct blow to the hand

Often caused by an athlete hitting a hard object with the fist

Symptoms
Pain localized around the injured area

Possibly a grating sensation

Signs
Swelling and deformity around the injured area

Loss of function

First Aid
Immobilize the hand and fingers.

Secure the hand to the body by applying an arm sling.

Treat for shock if necessary.

Gently apply ice over the area for 15 minutes.

Send the athlete to a physician or medical facility.

Playing Status
The athlete cannot return to activity until he or she is released by a physician and has normal wrist and hand strength, motion, and flexibility.

Prevention
Make sure athletes wear protective hand pads in football and hockey.

Finger Dislocation or Subluxation

Definition
The finger bone(s) moves out of position (see Figure 12.14).

Cause
Direct blow to the end of the finger

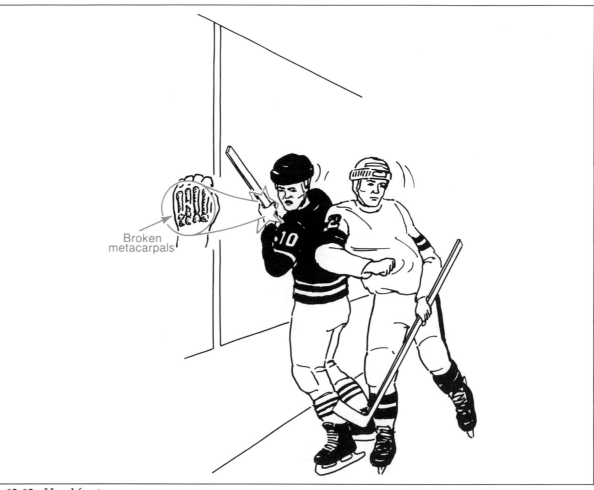

Figure 12.13 Hand fracture.

Symptom
The athlete may have heard a popping sound when the injury occurred.

Signs
Noticeable deformity

Possibly swelling

First Aid
Immobilize the finger in the position in which you found it.

Do not try to relocate the finger. It may also be fractured, and relocating it can displace the fracture and cause further injury.

Treat for shock if necessary.

Gently apply ice over the area for 15 minutes.

Send the athlete to a physician or an emergency medical facility.

Playing Status
The athlete cannot return to activity until he

or she is released by a physician and has normal grip strength and normal finger motion.

The athlete must use protective taping of the finger when he or she returns to activity.

Prevention
Tape vulnerable fingers before practice and competitions.

Finger Sprain (Jammed Finger)

Definition
This is a stretch or tear of the ligament(s) holding the finger bones together. If the sprain is severe, it can also tear off a piece of the bone (avulsion fracture).

Cause
Direct blow to the end of the finger

Signs
Swelling around the sprained joint

Loss of motion of the injured joint

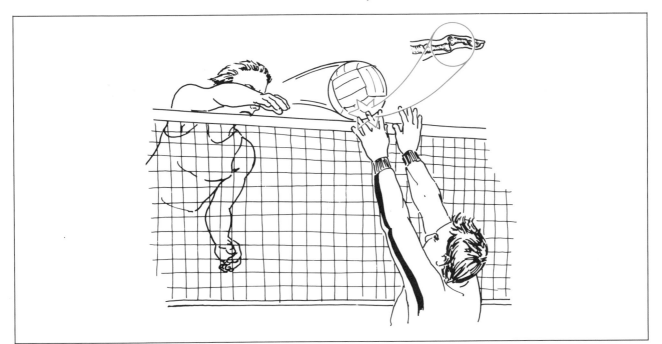

Figure 12.14 Finger dislocation.

Possibly a deformity around the joint

First Aid

Treat for shock if necessary.

Gently apply ice over the area for 15 minutes.

If pain and loss of motion are severe, immobilize the finger and send the athlete to a physician or emergency medical facility.

Playing Status

For Grade II and III sprains, the athlete cannot return to activity until he or she is released by a physician and has normal grip strength and finger motion.

The athlete must use protective taping of the finger when he or she returns to activity.

Prevention

Tape vulnerable fingers before practice and games.

Forearm, Wrist, and Hand Injury Summary

See Table 12.4 for a summary of how to care for the common forearm, wrist, and hand injuries in sport.

Although seemingly minor compared to life-threatening conditions and lower extremity injuries that prevent weight-bearing activity such as walking, upper extremity injuries can bring an end to athletes' careers in certain sports. Sports in which throwing, swinging, lifting, catching, pushing, or pulling are required demand intact shoulders, arms, wrists, and hands.

Hip and Thigh

Now we'll move down to the lower body and examine the common acute and chronic injuries that can occur to the hips, legs, and feet. You are well aware of the importance of healthy "wheels" to perform most sport activities. So read the next section closely to make sure your athletes can keep rolling along.

Acute Hip and Thigh Injuries

Hip injuries can be extremely painful and debilitating. And thigh injuries, especially muscle strains and contusions, are common to most sports. During the early season many athletes suffer strains to the quadriceps, hamstrings, and groin muscles of the thigh because they are out of shape with weak, inflexible muscles. In high school football, injuries to the thigh have been found to be the most common injury, accounting for 17.4% of all injuries (NATA, 1989a). The following section will help you to address the painful hip and prevalent thigh injuries your athletes

Table 12.4   First Aid Summary for Forearm, Wrist, and Hand Injuries

	Acute				
	Forearm fracture	Wrist sprain	Hand fracture	Finger dislocation/ subluxation	Finger sprain
Common evaluation findings					
Mechanism					
Sudden	X	X	X	X	X
Gradual					
Signs					
Swelling	X	G. II & III	X	X	X
Deformity	X	G. III	X	X	G. II & III
Discoloration	X	Possible	X	X	X
Warm to touch					
Muscle spasm	X	X	X	X	X
Tenderness to touch	X	X	X	X	X
Loss of motion	X	G. II & III	X	X	G. II & III
Symptoms					
Pain	X	X	X	X	X
Grating	X		X	X	
Numbness	X		X	X	
Popping	X	Possible	X	X	Possible
First aid					
PRICE	X	X	X	X	X
Immobilization	X	G. II & III	X	X	G. II & III
Monitor heart/breathing	X	G. II & III	X	X	G. II & III
Treat shock	X	G. II & III	X	X	G. II & III
Medical attention	X	X	X	X	X

X indicates that the evaluation or first aid applies to the problem.

G. = Grade

might experience. Note that only acute injuries are included, because in young athletes, these are more common than chronic hip and thigh problems.

Hip Contusion (Hip Pointer)

Definition
This is a bruise to the front, top of the hipbone (see Figure 12.15).

Cause
Direct blow to the front of the hipbone

History
The athlete was hit on the hipbone by another player.

The athlete fell or dove and hit the hipbone on the ground.

Signs
Inability to move the thigh forward

Possibly swelling and discoloration over the injury

First Aid
If pain and loss of function are severe, immobilize the hip and leg and send for emergency medical assistance.

Treat for shock if necessary.

Gently apply ice over the area for 15 minutes.

Playing Status
For moderate to severe contusions, the ath-

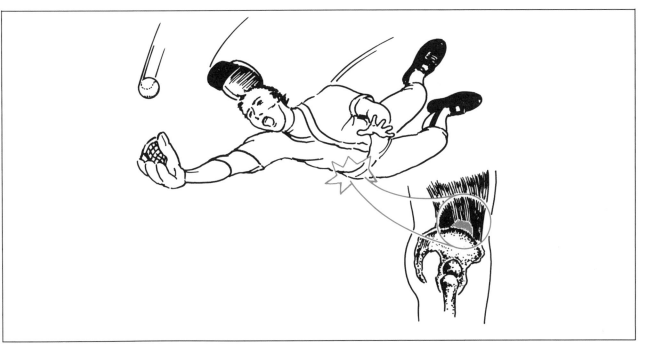

Figure 12.15 Hip contusion (hip pointer).

lete cannot return to activity until he or she is released by a physician and has normal hip and thigh strength and hip motion and flexibility.

The athlete should wear a protective pad over the hip once he or she returns to activity.

Prevention
Make sure athletes wear protective hip pads during football, volleyball, hockey, baseball, and softball participation.

Hip Flexor Strain

Definition
A stretch or tear of the hip flexor muscles, located high on the front of the thigh (see Figure 12.16).

Causes
Forceful contraction or stretch of the hip flexor muscle(s)

Weak or inflexible muscles are especially prone to strain.

History
The athlete complains of pain high on the front of the thigh.

The athlete was not hurt by a direct blow or a twisting injury.

The athlete may have heard a pop in a Grade III strain.

Signs
Possibly a deformity to the muscle

Possibly swelling and discoloration

First Aid
For a minor strain, gently stretch the hip flexor muscles (see Appendix B).

For moderate to severe strains where pain and loss of function are severe, prevent the athlete from walking on the injured leg and send him or her to a physician or emergency medical facility.

Treat for shock if necessary.

Gently apply ice over the area for 15 minutes.

Playing Status
For Grade II and III strains, the athlete cannot return to activity until he or she is released by a physician and has full hip flexor strength and flexibility.

The athlete may wear an elastic wrap or a commercial thigh sleeve to support the thigh when he or she returns to activity.

Prevention
Have athletes undergo preseason strength and flexibility training.

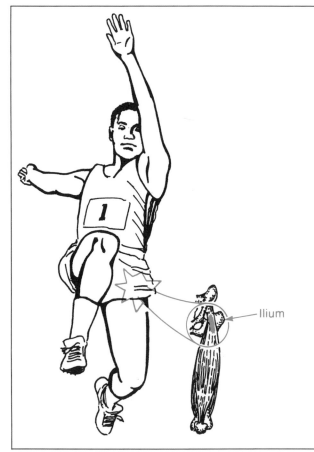

Figure 12.16 Hip flexor strain.

Make sure athletes do an adequate warm-up, including stretching, before activity.

Adductor Strain

Definition
This is a stretch or tear of the adductor (inside thigh) muscle(s).

Causes
Forceful contraction or stretch of the adductor muscle(s)

Weak or inflexible muscles are especially prone to strain.

History
The athlete complains of pain on the inside of the thigh and may have heard or felt a pop.

The athlete was not hurt by a direct blow or a twisting injury.

The athlete may have heard or felt a pop.

Signs
Inability to move the thigh inward toward the other thigh

Possibly a deformity at the site of the injury

Possibly swelling and discoloration

First Aid
For a minor strain, have the athlete gently stretch the adductor muscles (see Appendix B).

For Grade II or III strains where there is severe pain or loss of function, prevent the athlete from walking on the injured leg, and send him or her to a physician or an emergency medical facility.

Treat for shock if necessary.

Gently apply ice over the area for 15 minutes.

Playing Status
For Grade II and III strains, the athlete cannot return to activity until he or she is released by a physician and has normal adductor strength and flexibility.

The athlete may wear an elastic wrap or a commercial thigh sleeve to support the thigh when he or she returns to activity.

Prevention
Have athletes undergo preseason strength and flexibility training.

Make sure athletes do an adequate warm-up, including stretching, before activity.

Thigh Fracture

Definition
This is a break of the thighbone (femur), such as that shown in Figure 12.17.

Causes
Direct blow to the thigh

Twisting or torsion injury of the thigh

Symptoms
The athlete may have heard a pop or snap.

The athlete may complain of a grating feeling.

There is pain at the injury site when the thigh above and below the injury is gently squeezed.

Signs
Muscle spasm

Possibly a deformity at the site of the injury

First Aid
Send for emergency medical assistance.

Immobilize the entire leg and hip in the position in which you found it.

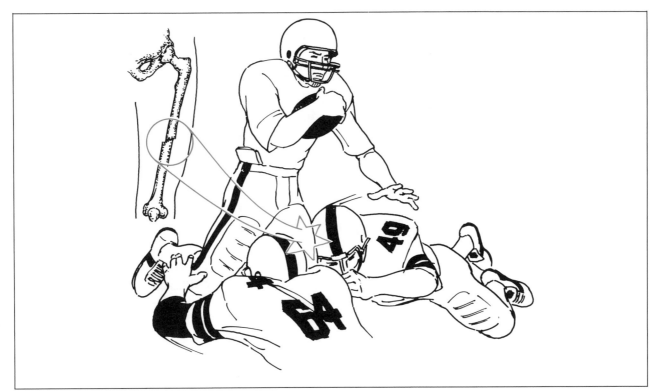

Figure 12.17 Thigh fracture.

Secure the leg to the other leg with an ace wrap.

Treat for shock if necessary.

Gently apply ice over the area for 15 minutes.

Playing Status
The athlete cannot return to activity until he or she is released by a physician.

The athlete must wear a protective pad over the thigh when he or she returns to activity.

Prevention
Make sure athletes wear protective thigh pads in football and hockey.

Thigh Contusion

Definition
This is a bruise to the soft tissues or bones of the thigh.

Cause
Direct blow to the thigh

Symptom
Pain over the contused area

Signs
Possibly muscle spasm

Possibly swelling

First Aid
If pain and loss of motion are severe, immobilize the entire injured leg and hip, and send for emergency medical assistance.

Treat for shock if necessary.

Gently apply ice over the area for 15 minutes while the knee is bent.

Playing Status
For moderate to severe contusions, the athlete cannot return to activity until he or she is released by a physician and has normal knee motion and flexibility and thigh muscle strength.

The athlete must wear a protective pad over the thigh when she or he returns to activity.

Prevention
Make sure athletes wear thigh pads in football and hockey.

Quadricep Strain

Definition
This is a stretch or tear of the quadricep muscle(s), similar to that shown in Figure 12.18.

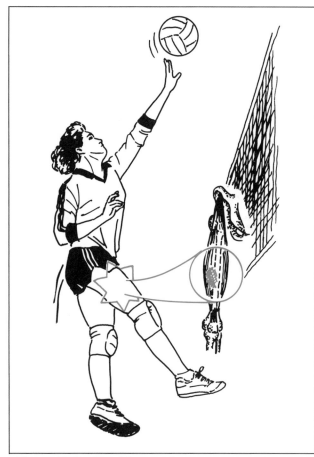

Figure 12.18 Quadricep strain.

Causes
Forceful contraction or stretch of the quad muscle(s)

Weak or inflexible muscles are especially prone to strain.

History
The athlete complains of pain in the front of the thigh.

The athlete was not hurt by a direct blow or a twisting injury.

Signs
Possibly a deformity in the muscle (Grade III)

Possibly swelling and discoloration

First Aid
For mild strains where pain and loss of function is minimal, have the athlete gently stretch the quad muscles (see Appendix B).

For moderate to severe strains, prevent the athlete from walking on the injured leg, and send him or her to a physician or an emergency medical facility.

Treat for shock if necessary.

Gently apply ice over the area for 15 minutes.

Playing Status
For Grade II and III sprains, the athlete cannot return to activity until he or she is released by a physician.

The athlete must have normal quadricep strength and flexibility and normal knee and hip motion.

The athlete may wear an elastic wrap or a commercial thigh sleeve to support the thigh when he or she returns to activity.

Prevention
Have athletes undergo preseason strength and flexibility training.

Make sure athletes do an adequate warm-up, including stretching, before activity.

Hamstring Strain

Definition
This is a stretch or tear of the hamstring muscle(s) (see Figure 12.19).

Causes
Forceful contraction or stretch of the hamstring muscle(s)

Weak or inflexible muscles are especially prone to strain.

History
The athlete complains of pain in the back of the thigh.

The athlete was not hurt by a direct blow or a twisting injury.

The athlete may have heard or felt a pop.

Signs
Possibly a deformity at the site of the injury

Possibly swelling and discoloration

First Aid
For minor strains, have the athlete gently stretch the hamstring muscles (see Appendix B).

For Grade II and III strains where pain and loss of function are severe, prevent the athlete from walking on the injured leg, and send him or her to a physician or an emergency medical facility.

Treat for shock if necessary.

Gently apply ice over the area for 15 minutes.

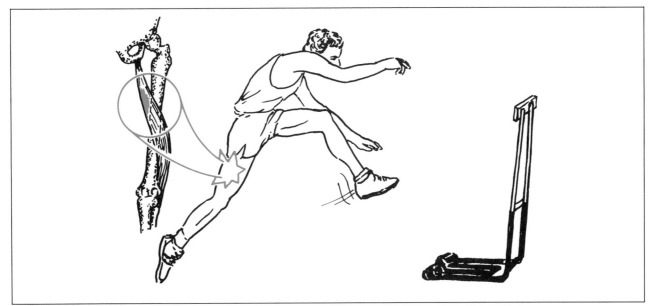

Figure 12.19 Hamstring strain.

Playing Status
For Grade II and III strains, the athlete cannot return to activity until he or she is released by a physician and has normal hamstring strength and flexibility.

The athlete may wear an elastic wrap or a commercial thigh sleeve to support the thigh when he or she returns to activity.

Prevention
Have athletes undergo preseason strength and flexibility training.

Make sure athletes do an adequate warm-up, including stretching, before activity.

Hip and Thigh Injury Summary

An athlete generates a lot of power from the waist to the knees. It is not surprising, then, that this part of the body is often injured. Table 12.5 will serve as a handy reference to help you properly care for your athletes' hip and thigh injuries.

Knee

The knee is probably the second-most-commonly injured area in all of sport. In high school football, wrestling, and boys' basketball, knee injuries occur at a 14.5%, 15%, and 10% rate, respectively, among all injuries (NATA, 1989a, 1989b). Knee injuries occur at an even higher rate (18%) among high school girl basketball players (NATA, 1989b). So it's apparent that you should know how to provide first aid for acute and chronic knee conditions that your athletes experience.

Acute Knee Injuries

Knee Sprain

Definition
This is a stretch or tear of the ligament(s) that hold the knee bones in place (see Figure 12.20).

Causes
Direct blow to either the front, side, or back of the knee

Twisting or torsion injury to the knee

Hyperextension or hyperflexion injury to the knee

Weak thigh muscles make an athlete especially prone to sprains.

History
The athlete was hurt by a direct blow, a twisting injury, or a hyperflexion or hyperextension injury.

The athlete may have heard or felt a pop.

Signs
Possibly swelling and discoloration

Table 12.5   First Aid Summary for Hip and Thigh Injuries

	Acute						
	Hip contusion	Hip flexor strain	Adductor strain	Thigh bone (femur) fracture	Thigh contusion	Quadricep strain	Hamstring strain
Common evaluation findings							
Mechanism							
Sudden	X	X	X	X	X	X	X
Gradual		X	X			X	X
Signs							
Swelling	X	G. II & III	G. II & III	X	X	G. II & III	G. II & III
Deformity	Possible	G. III	G. III	X		G. III	G. III
Discoloration	X	G. II & III	G. II & III	X	X	G. II & III	G. II & III
Warm to touch							
Muscle spasm	X	X	X	X	X	X	X
Tenderness to touch	X	X	X	X	X	X	X
Loss of motion	X	G. II & III	G. II & III	X	X	G. II & III	G. II & III
Symptoms							
Pain	X	X	X	X	X	X	X
Grating	X			X	X		
Numbness	Possible			Possible	Possible		
Popping		Possible	Possible	X		Possible	Possible
First aid							
PRICE	X	X	X	X	X	X	X
Immobilization	G. II & III	G. III	G. III	X	G. II & III	G. III	G. III
Monitor heart/breathing	G. II & III	G. III	G. III	X	G. II & III	G. III	G. III
Treat shock	G. II & III	G. III	G. III	X	G. II & III	G. III	G. III
Medical attention	X	X	X	X	X	X	X

X indicates that the evaluation or first aid applies to the problem.

G. = Grade

Possibly an inability to bend or straighten the knee

Possibly inability to walk without limping

First Aid

If pain and loss of function are severe (Grade II and III sprains), prevent the athlete from walking on the injured leg, and send him or her to a physician or an emergency medical facility.

In Grade II and III sprains, splint the knee in the most comfortable position.

Treat for shock if necessary.

Gently apply ice over the area for 15 minutes.

Playing Status

For severe pain and loss of function, the athlete cannot return to activity until he or she is released by a physician and has normal knee strength and motion.

Prevention

Have athletes undergo preseason strength and flexibility training.

Dislocated or Subluxated Patella (Kneecap)

Definition

The kneecap slips out of the groove on the upper thighbone (see Figure 12.21).

Causes

Direct blow to the inside of the kneecap

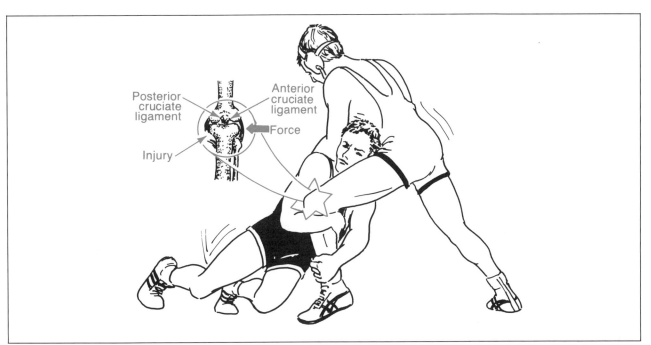

Figure 12.20 Knee sprain.

Forceful contraction of the outside quadricep muscle(s)

Twisting or torsion injury to the knee

Weak inside quadricep muscle can leave the athlete prone to kneecap dislocation or subluxation.

History
The athlete may have heard or felt a pop.

Symptom
Feeling of the kneecap going out of place

Signs
Possibly the kneecap displaced to the outside of the knee

Possibly swelling

Possibly an inability to bend or straighten the knee

First Aid
If the kneecap is still displaced, send for emergency medical assistance, and immobilize the knee and entire leg.

Do not attempt to relocate a dislocated kneecap.

If the kneecap is back in place, prevent the athlete from walking on the injured leg, and send him or her to a physician or an emergency medical facility.

Treat for shock if necessary.

Gently apply ice over the area for 15 minutes.

Playing Status
The athlete cannot return to activity until he or she is released by a physician and has normal knee strength and motion.

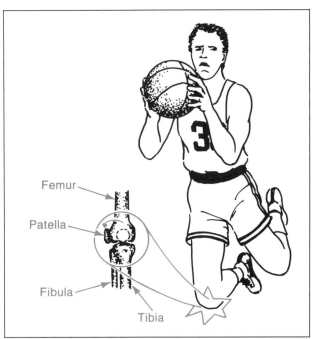

Figure 12.21 Dislocated patella (kneecap).

The athlete should wear a patellar stabilizing brace when he or she returns to activity.

Prevention
Have athletes undergo preseason strength and flexibility training.

Cartilage Tear

Definition
This is a tear of the cartilage on the lower leg bone (see Figure 12.22).

Causes
Direct blow to the knee

Twisting or torsion injury to the knee, especially while the knee is bent

History
The athlete complains that his or her knee locks or won't move.

The athlete complains of the knee giving out.

Symptom
Pain at the injury site, especially along the joint line between the upper and lower leg bones.

Signs
Possibly an inability to completely bend or straighten the knee

Possibly delayed swelling (cartilage injury alone) or immediate swelling (cartilage injury and ligament sprain)

First Aid
Cartilage tears commonly occur with severe knee sprains, so if pain and loss of function are severe, prevent the athlete from walking on the injured leg, splint the knee in a comfortable position, and send him or her to a physician or an emergency medical facility.

Treat for shock if necessary.

Gently apply ice over the area for 15 minutes.

Playing Status
The athlete cannot return to activity until he or she is released by a physician and has normal knee strength and motion.

Prevention
Have athletes undergo preseason strength and flexibility training.

Chronic Knee Injuries

Osgood-Schlatter disease

Definition
There is inflammation where the quadricep tendon inserts into the lower leg bone (see Figure 12.23). This occurs in young and growing athletes.

Causes
Forceful contraction of the quadricep muscle(s)

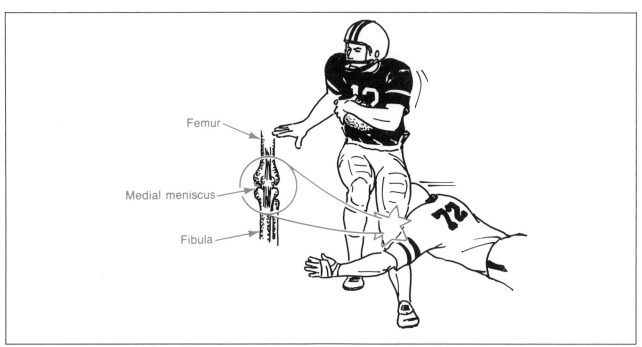

Figure 12.22 Cartilage tear.

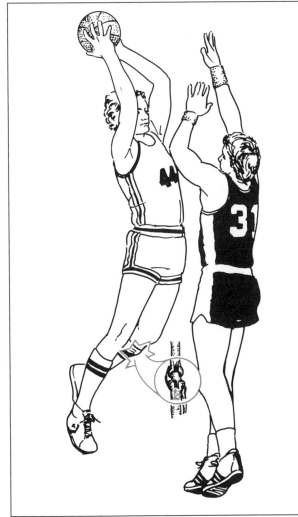

Figure 12.23 Osgood-Schlatter disease.

Weak or inflexible thigh muscles can contribute to this injury.

History
The athlete was not hurt by a twisting injury.

Symptoms
Pain below the knee at the top of the lower leg bone

Pain over area if bumped

Signs
Inability to forcefully straighten the knee, especially when jumping and lifting weights

A bump below the knee, on the lower leg

First Aid
If pain and loss of motion are severe, prevent the athlete from walking on the injured leg, and send him or her to a physician or an emergency medical facility.

For pain and loss of motion that are mild, have the athlete rest the knee until he or she is seen and released by a physician.

Treat for shock if necessary.

Gently apply ice over the area for 15 minutes.

Playing Status
The athlete cannot return to activity until he or she is released by a physician and is pain-free.

The athlete should also stretch the hamstring and calf muscles daily (see Appendix B) when he or she returns to activity.

The athlete should wear a knee pad to protect the area from direct blows.

Prevention
Have athletes undergo preseason strength and flexibility training.

Make sure athletes do an adequate warm-up, including stretching, before activity.

Patellar Tendinitis

Definition
This is an inflammation of the tendon that attaches the kneecap to the lower leg bone (see Figure 12.24).

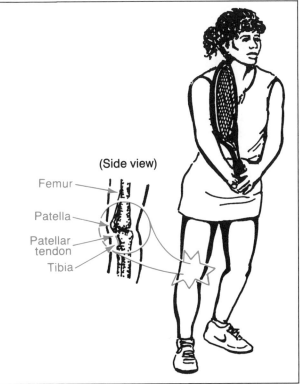

Figure 12.24 Patellar tendinitis.

Causes
Forceful contraction of the quadricep muscle(s)

Weak or inflexible thigh muscles can contribute to this injury.

History
The athlete was not hurt by a direct blow or a twisting injury.

Symptoms
Pain below the kneecap

Pain with running and jumping activities

Signs
Inability to forcefully straighten the knee, especially during jumping or weight lifting

Possibly swelling below the kneecap

First Aid
If pain and loss of function are severe, prevent the athlete from walking on the injured leg, and send him or her to a physician or an emergency medical facility.

If pain and loss of function are mild, have the athlete rest the knee until he or she is seen and released by a physician.

Treat for shock if necessary.

Gently apply ice over the area for 15 minutes.

Playing Status
The athlete cannot return to activity until he or she is released by a physician and movement is pain-free.

The athlete should also stretch the hamstring, quadricep, and calf muscles daily (see Appendix B) when he or she returns to activity.

The athlete may wear a rubberized neoprene knee sleeve to keep the knee warm during activity.

Prevention
Have athletes undergo preseason strength and flexibility training.

Make sure athletes do an adequate warm-up, including stretching, before activity.

Patellofemoral Joint Pain

Definition
This is an inflammation or irritation of the tissues under the kneecap and on the thighbone area around the kneecap.

Causes
Direct blow to the top of the kneecap

Inability of the kneecap to properly track in the groove in the thighbone

Repeated episodes of patellar (kneecap) dislocation and subluxation

Weak or inflexible quadriceps or hamstring muscles can contribute to this injury.

History
The athlete may have previously suffered from a blow to the kneecap or from a dislocated or subluxated kneecap.

Symptoms
Pain with running, jumping, or stair climbing

Pain behind the kneecap

A grating feeling behind the kneecap

Achiness while sitting for extended periods

First Aid
If pain and loss of function are severe, prevent the athlete from walking on the injured leg, and send him or her to a physician or an emergency medical facility.

If pain and loss of function are mild, have the athlete rest the knee until he or she is seen and released by a physician.

Treat for shock if necessary.

Gently apply ice over the area for 15 minutes.

Playing Status
The athlete cannot return to activity until he or she is released by a physician, is pain-free, and has normal quadricep strength.

The athlete should also stretch the hamstring, quadricep, and calf muscles daily (see Appendix B) when he or she returns to activity.

The athlete may wear a rubberized neoprene knee sleeve to keep the knee warm during activity.

Prevention
Have athletes undergo preseason strength and flexibility training.

Make sure athletes do an adequate warm-up, including stretching, before activity.

Iliotibial Band Strain

Definition
This is a stretch or irritation of the connective tissue along the outside of the thigh (see Figure 12.25).

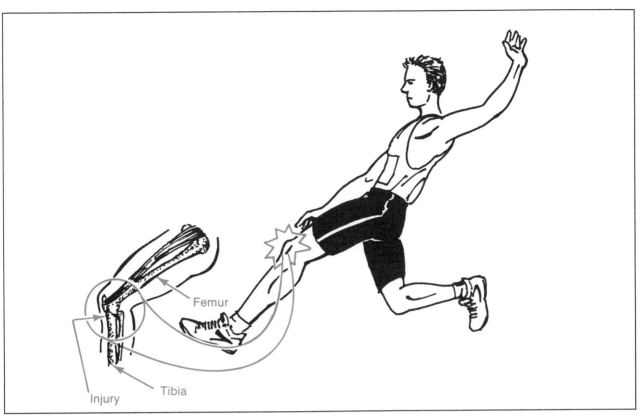

Figure 12.25 Iliotibial band strain.

Causes
Forceful stretch of the connective tissue that attaches to the outside of the knee

Weak or inflexible thigh muscles

History
The athlete was not hurt by a direct blow or a twisting injury.

Symptoms
Pain along the outside of the knee

Pain with running or jumping

Sign
Possibly swelling

First Aid
If pain and loss of motion are severe, prevent the athlete from walking on the injured leg, and send him or her to a physician or an emergency medical facility.

If pain and loss of motion are mild, have the athlete rest the knee until he or she is seen and released by a physician.

Treat for shock if necessary.

Gently apply ice over the area for 15 minutes.

Playing Status
The athlete cannot return to activity until he or she is released by a physician and is pain-free.

The athlete should also stretch the iliotibial band, hamstrings, and quadriceps daily (see Appendix B) when he or she returns to activity.

The athlete may wear a rubberized neoprene knee sleeve to keep the knee warm during activity.

Prevention
Have athletes undergo preseason strength and flexibility training.

Make sure athletes do an adequate warm-up, including stretching, before activity.

Knee Injury Summary

The joint that allows for lower leg movement, so important in sport activities, is also one of the most frequently injured. Refer to Table 12.6 if you have any questions about the proper care for common knee injuries in sport.

Table 12.6   First Aid Summary for Knee Injuries

	Acute			Chronic			
	Sprain	Dislocated/ subluxated kneecap	Cartilage tear	Osgood Schlatter	Patellar tendinitis	Patellofemoral joint pain	Iliotibial band strain
Common evaluation findings							
Mechanism							
Sudden	X	X	X				
Gradual				X	X	X	X
Signs							
Swelling	X	X	Often delayed	X	Possible	Possible	
Deformity		X		X			
Discoloration	Possible	Possible	Possible	Possible	Possible		
Warm to touch							
Muscle spasm	X	X	Possible				Possible
Tenderness to touch	X	X	X	X	X	X	X
Loss of motion	G. II & III	X	X	If severe	If severe	If severe	If severe
Symptoms							
Pain	X	X	X	X	X	X	X
Grating		X	X			X	
Numbness		Possible					
Popping	X	X	X			X	
First aid							
PRICE	X	X	X	X	X	X	X
Immobilization	G. II & III	X	If severe	If severe	If severe	If severe	If severe
Monitor heart/breathing	G. II & III	X	If severe				
Treat shock	G. II & III	X	If severe				
Medical attention	X	X	X	X	X	X	X

X indicates that the evaluation or first aid applies to the problem.

G. = Grade

Lower Leg, Ankle, and Foot

In addition to knee injuries, ankle and foot injuries are also quite common in sport. The ankle and foot are the most commonly injured body parts in high school girls' and boys' basketball (NATA, 1989b). Among all types of injuries, ankle and foot problems account for 41% and 32%, respectively, of athletes' physical setbacks. And in high school football (NATA, 1989a) the ankle alone was the site of 16% of all injuries. Obviously, it is crucial that you learn how to care for these lower extremity injuries.

Acute Lower Leg and Ankle Injuries

Calf Strain

Definition
This is a stretch or tear of the calf muscle(s) (see Figure 12.26).

Causes
Forceful contraction of the calf muscle(s)

Weak or inflexible muscles are especially prone to strain.

History
The athlete was not hurt by a direct blow or a twisting injury.

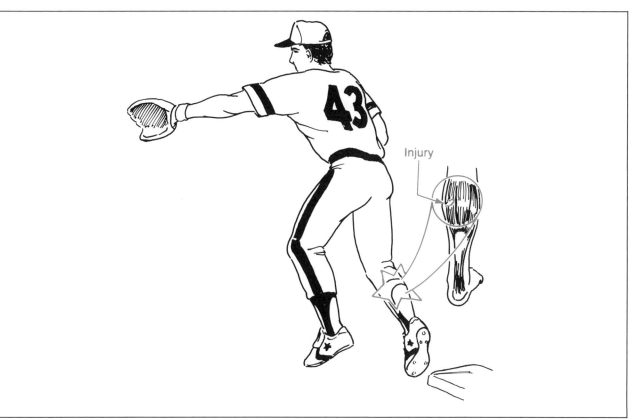

Figure 12.26 Calf strain.

The athlete may have performed an explosive move such as jumping or sprinting quickly.

Symptom
Pain in the back of the calf

Signs
Possibly swelling and discoloration if the injury is severe

Possibly a deformity at the site of injury.

Possibly an inability to point the foot without pain

First Aid
For a minor strain, have the athlete gently stretch the calf muscles (see Appendix B).

If pain and loss of function are severe, prevent the athlete from walking on the injured leg, and send him or her to a physician or an emergency medical facility.

Treat for shock if necessary.

Gently apply ice over the area for 15 minutes.

Playing Status
The athlete cannot return to activity until he or she is released by a physician and has normal calf strength and flexibility.

The athlete may wear an elastic wrap or a commercial calf sleeve to support the calf when he or she returns to activity.

Prevention
Have athletes undergo preseason strength and flexibility training.

Make sure athletes do an adequate warm-up, including stretching, before activity.

Lower Leg Contusion

Definition
This is a bruise to the lower leg, such as the one shown in Figure 12.27.

Cause
Direct blow

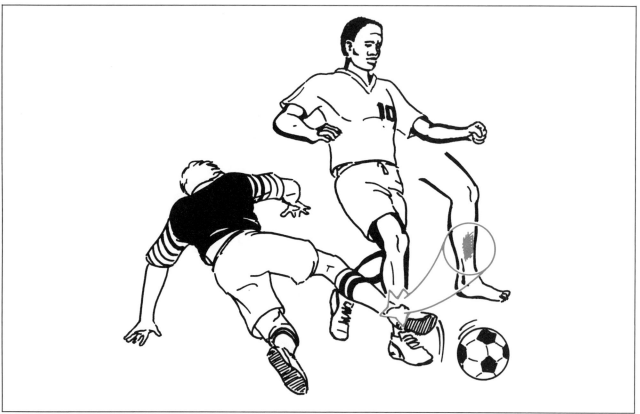

Figure 12.27 Lower leg contusion.

Symptoms
Pain over the contused area

Possibly numbness or tingling in the foot if the swelling compresses the nerves and arteries to the foot

Signs
Possibly an inability to bend the knee or point the foot down

Swelling and discoloration

First Aid
If pain and loss of motion are severe, prevent the athlete from walking on the injured leg, and send him or her to a physician or an emergency medical facility.

If it is a severe contusion over a bone, splint the lower leg and knee.

Treat for shock if necessary.

Gently apply ice over the area for 15 minutes.

Playing Status
For moderate to severe contusions, the athlete cannot return to activity until he or she is released by a physician and has normal lower leg strength and flexibility.

The athlete should wear a protective pad when he or she returns to activity.

Prevention
Make sure athletes wear protective padding during soccer and baseball or softball.

Ankle Sprain

Definition
This is a stretch or tear of the ligament(s) holding the ankle bones together.

In an inversion sprain, the foot rolls in and damages the outside ankle ligaments and sometimes the inside ligaments (see Figure 12.28). This is the most common ankle sprain.

In an eversion sprain, the foot rolls out and damages the inside ankle ligaments and sometimes the outside ligaments

Causes
Direct blow to the ankle

Twisting or torsion injury to the ankle

History
The athlete landed on another athlete's foot.

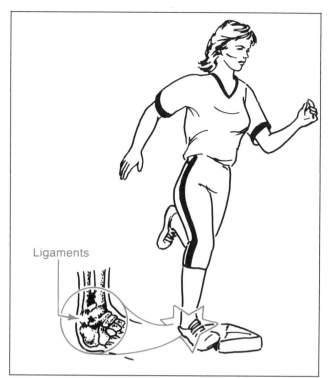

Figure 12.28   Inversion ankle sprain.

Prevention
Have athletes undergo preseason strength and flexibility training.

Chronic Lower Leg, Ankle, and Foot Injuries

Shinsplints

Definition
This is a stretch, tear, or irritation of the shin muscle(s), tendon(s), or bone covering (see Figure 12.29).

Causes
Forceful contraction or stretch of the shin muscle(s)

Repetitive pounding of the feet on hard surfaces such as concrete

Weak or inflexible muscles are especially prone to strain.

The athlete tripped in a hole or caught a cleat on the playing surface.

The athlete may have heard or felt a pop.

Symptom
Pain around the inside and/or outside ankle bones

Signs
Swelling

Possibly discoloration

First Aid
If pain, swelling, and loss of motion are severe, prevent the athlete from walking on the ankle. Immobilize the ankle and send the athlete to a physician or an emergency medical facility.

Treat for shock if necessary.

Gently apply ice over the area for 15 minutes.

Playing Status
The athlete cannot return to activity until he or she is released by a physician and has normal ankle strength, motion, and flexibility.

The athlete should use protective tape or a brace when he or she returns to activity.

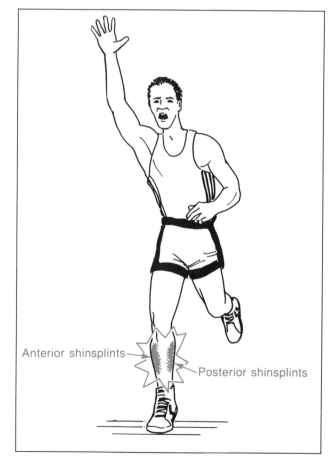

Figure 12.29   Shinsplints.

Flat arches, which fail to absorb shock, allow shock to be transmitted up the lower leg bone.

History
The athlete was not hurt by a direct blow or a twisting injury.

The athlete participates in a repetitive, stressful activity such as running or aerobic dance.

Symptoms
Pain along the shin

Pain with running and jumping activities

Signs
Possibly swelling

Possibly an inability to run or jump

First Aid
If pain and loss of motion are severe, prevent the athlete from walking on the injured leg, and send him or her to a physician or an emergency medical facility.

For minor shinsplints, have the athlete gently stretch the calf muscles (see Appendix B).

Gently apply ice over the area for 15 minutes.

If moderate to mild pain persists for more than 2 weeks, send the athlete to a physician to rule out a possible stress fracture.

Playing Status
In severe or prolonged (several weeks) cases of shinsplints, the athlete cannot return to activity until he or she is released by a physician and is pain-free.

The athlete should perform calf stretches and ankle-strengthening exercises when he or she is able to return to activity.

The athlete may wear arch supports or tape and/or an elastic wrap or a commercial calf sleeve to support the shin when he or she returns to activity.

Prevention
Have athletes undergo preseason strength and flexibility training.

Make sure athletes do an adequate warm-up, including stretching, before activity.

Achilles Tendinitis

Definition
This is a stretch, tear, or irritation to the tendon that attaches the calf muscles to the heel (see Figure 12.30).

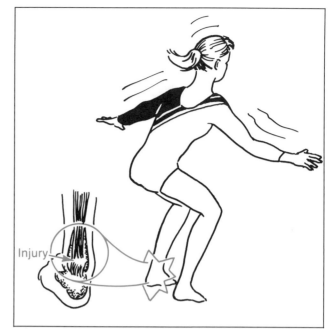

Figure 12.30 Achilles tendinitis.

Causes
Forceful contraction or stretch of the calf muscle(s)

Weak or inflexible muscles are especially prone to strain.

History
The athlete was not hurt by a direct blow or a twisting injury.

The athlete participates in a repetitive, stressful activity that requires going up on the toes (gymnastics, basketball, volleyball, etc.)

Symptoms
Pain just above the heel

Pain with running and jumping

Signs
Inability to point the foot down

Possibly swelling

First Aid
For minor Achilles tendinitis, have the athlete gently stretch the calf muscles (see Appendix B).

If pain and loss of motion are severe, prevent the athlete from walking on the injured leg, and send him or her to a physician or an emergency medical facility.

Treat for shock if necessary.

Gently apply ice over the area for 15 minutes.

Playing Status

The athlete cannot return to activity until he or she is released by a physician and is pain-free.

The athlete should strengthen and stretch the Achilles tendon when he or she returns to activity.

The athlete may wear heel lifts or heel cups in the shoes when he or she returns to activity.

Prevention

Have athletes undergo preseason strength and flexibility training.

Make sure athletes do an adequate warm-up, including stretching, before activity.

Heel Bruise

Definition

This is a bruise to the muscle, bone, and soft tissues of the heel.

Causes

Wearing shoes with little heel cushioning

Exercising on hard surfaces such as concrete

History

The athlete was not hurt by a direct blow or a twisting injury.

Symptoms

Heel pain

Pain with running or jumping

Sign

Inability to land or walk on the injured heel

First Aid

If pain and loss of motion are severe, prevent the athlete from walking on the injured leg, and send him or her to a physician or an emergency medical facility.

Treat for shock if necessary.

Gently apply ice over the area for 15 minutes.

Playing Status

For moderate to severe heel bruises, the athlete cannot return to activity until he or she is released by a physician and is pain-free.

The athlete should wear shock-absorbing heel cushions to protect the heel when he or she returns to activity.

Prevention

Make sure athletes wear shoes with plenty of heel cushioning.

Plantar Fasciitis

Definition

This is a stretching or inflammation of the tissue that connects to the heel and toes (see Figure 12.31).

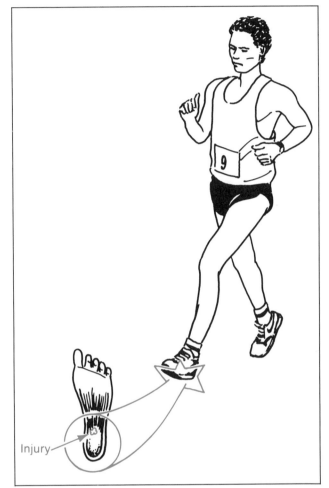

Figure 12.31   Plantar fasciitis.

Causes

Forceful contraction or stretch of the calf muscle(s)

Flat feet

Wearing shoes with inadequate arch support

Weak or inflexible muscles are especially prone to strain.

History

The athlete was not hurt by a direct blow or a twisting injury.

Symptoms

Pain along the arch or near the bottom of the heel

Feeling of muscle tightness or weakness

Signs
The arch may flatten out.

Inability to push off with the foot or point the foot down.

Possibly an inability to walk without limping.

First Aid
For minor plantar fasciitis, have the athlete gently stretch the calf muscles and plantar fascia (see Appendix B).

If pain and loss of function are severe, prevent the athlete from walking on the injured leg, and send him or her to a physician or an emergency medical facility.

Playing Status
For moderate to severe plantar fasciitis, the athlete cannot return to activity until he or she is released by a physician and is pain-free.

The athlete should continue calf and plantar fascia stretches once he or she returns to activity.

The athlete may wear heel cushions or arch inserts to support the arch when he or she returns to activity.

Prevention
Have athletes undergo preseason strength and flexibility training.

Make sure athletes do an adequate warm-up, including stretching, before activity.

Table 12.7   First Aid Summary for Lower Leg, Shin, Ankle, and Foot Injuries

	Acute			Chronic			
	Calf strain	Lower leg contusion	Ankle sprain	Shinsplints	Achilles tendinitis	Heel bruise	Plantar fasciitis
Common evaluation findings							
Mechanism							
Sudden	X	X	X			X	
Gradual	X			X	X	X	X
Signs							
Swelling	G. II & III	X	X		If severe		
Deformity	G. II & III	X	X				
Discoloration	G. II & III	X	X				
Warm to touch			Possible				
Muscle spasm	X	X	X		Possible		Possible
Tenderness to touch	X	X	X	X	X	X	X
Loss of motion	G. II & III	If severe	G. II & III	If severe	If severe	If severe	If severe
Symptoms							
Pain	X	X	X	X	X	X	X
Grating							
Numbness		Possible					
Popping			X				
First aid							
PRICE	X	X	X	X	X	X	X
Immobilization	If severe	If severe	X	If severe			
Monitor heart/breathing	If severe	If severe	X				
Treat shock	If severe	If severe	X				
Medical attention	X	X	X	X	X	X	X

X indicates that the evaluation or first aid applies to the problem.

G. = Grade

Lower Leg, Ankle, and Foot Injury Summary

Because of the prevalence of calf, shin, ankle, and foot injuries in sport, you'll want to be well versed in first aid techniques for the injuries presented. These common injuries and their appropriate care are summarized in Table 12.7.

Sport First Aid Recap

1. Musculoskeletal injuries are the most common types of injuries suffered by athletes.

2. It is important to understand the causes and implications of the three levels of injury severity—acute mild, acute Grade II and III, and chronic—in order to provide appropriate first aid treatment.

3. PRICE is beneficial for almost all types of musculoskeletal injuries.

4. Athletes with musculoskeletal injuries should not be allowed to return to activity unless they have been released by a physician and they have regained full motion, strength, and flexibility at the injured area.

CHAPTER 13

Soft-Tissue Injuries of the Face and Head

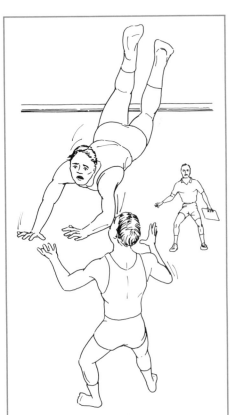

Andy Scott is helping to spot Greg Duncan on the high bar. Just as Greg prepares for his dismount, his right hand loses its grip, and he falls to the ground. Trying to cushion Greg's fall, Andy steps in. Unfortunately, he gets the worse end of the fall and catches an elbow from Greg right across the nose. His nose is bleeding heavily from the nostrils. How would you treat Andy's injury?

Trying to handle a bleeding face wound or any other head injury can be frightening. There's often so much blood that you can't see what you're doing; it may seem like the athlete is going to bleed to death.

When you encounter such situations, just remember that head and facial cuts generally look worse than they really are. The face and head have an extensive network of blood vessels. Therefore, a face or head injury may bleed a lot but in itself may not be extensive.

From Facial Cuts to Chipped Teeth

In this chapter you'll learn about the more common facial injuries and their care. We'll start with facial cuts, then examine typical injuries to the eyes, ears, nose, and mouth.

Most of these injuries should be seen by a physician, because they do involve a highly visible and important part of the body: the head. But if a physician or other medical professional is not present when a soft-tissue head injury occurs, you'll be glad that you learned the first aid information found in the remainder of this chapter.

Facial Laceration

Definition
This is a cut on the face, usually around the eyebrow (see Figure 13.1), chin, forehead, or nose.

151

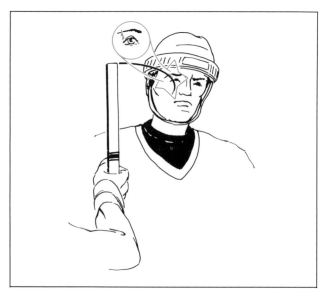

Figure 13.1   Facial laceration.

Cause
Usually a direct blow with an object such as a ball, elbow, racket, and the like

Symptom
Pain

Signs
Rapid bleeding

Possibly bruising of the skin

First Aid
Cover the injury with sterile gauze and apply pressure.

You can also close the injury with butterfly strips after bleeding stops, then cover with gauze.

Send the athlete to a physician.

Playing Status
The athlete cannot return to activity until he or she is released by a physician.

Prevention
Make sure athletes wear protective face masks and goggles when appropriate.

Black Eye

Definition
This is a contusion to the soft tissues around the eye.

Cause
Direct blow

Symptom
Pain

Signs
Swelling

Discoloration

A severe eye contusion may cause bleeding into the white of the eye or deformity, indicating a possible fracture of the bones around the eye.

First Aid
Rest

Ice

Send the athlete to a physician.

Playing Status
The athlete cannot return to activity until he or she is released by a physician.

Prevention
Make sure athletes wear protective eye goggles or shields.

Eye Laceration

Definition
This is a scratch to the cornea covering the eye.

Cause
The cornea is scratched by dirt, sand, glass, or other material that has gotten into the eye.

History
The athlete complains of something in the eye.

Symptoms
Pain

Burning sensation

Signs
Red, watery eye

Possibly swelling

Possibly a foreign object in the eye

Decreased vision

Blurred vision

Sensitivity to light

Possibly a scratch or cut on the eye

First Aid
Try to remove any small irritating particle such as dirt or glass, as shown in Figure 13.2.

Cover both eyes with sterile gauze. Otherwise, movements of the uninjured eye would cause the injured eye to move.

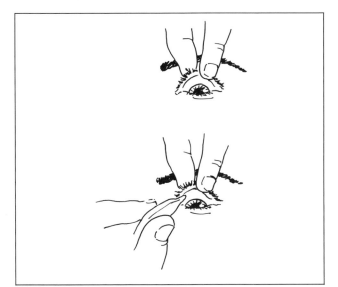

Figure 13.2 Removing a foreign particle from the eye.

Have the athlete rest in a semireclining position.

Send the athlete to a physician.

Playing Status
The athlete cannot return to activity until he or she is released by a physician.

Prevention
Make sure athletes wear protective eyeglasses, goggles, or shields.

For Eye Lacerations

DO NOT . . .

. . . rub the eye.
. . . try to remove embedded objects.
. . . try to remove contact lenses.
. . . try to wash the eye.

Ear Avulsion

Definition
This is a tear of the ear tissue, usually around the earlobe.

Cause
Sheer or tearing force on the ear

History
The athlete had an earring ripped out of the ear.

Symptom
Pain

Signs
Bleeding

Tear in the soft tissue of the ear

First Aid
Cover the injury with sterile gauze.

Apply direct pressure.

You can also apply ice if the bleeding doesn't stop.

Send the athlete to a physician.

If a piece of the ear is completely torn away, place it in sterile gauze and take it to the physician.

Playing Status
The athlete cannot return to activity until he or she is released by a physician.

Prevention
Forbid athletes to wear jewelry during activity.

Require athletes to wear protective headgear when appropriate.

Ear Contusion (Cauliflower Ear)

Definition
This is a contusion to the ear (see Figure 13.3).

Causes
Direct blow

Repeated rubbing of the ear against a hard surface

History
The athlete suffered a direct hit or repeated blows to the ear.

Symptoms
Pain

Possibly a burning feeling

Signs
Swelling of the outer ear

Discoloration

Warm feeling in ear

Redness

Deformity

First Aid
Apply ice over the injury.

Send the athlete to a physician.

Playing Status
The athlete cannot return to activity until he or she is released by a physician.

Prevention
Require athletes to wear protective headgear when appropriate.

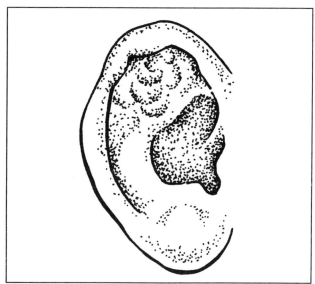

Figure 13.3   Ear contusion.

Broken Nose

Definition
This is a break in the cartilage or bone of the nose.

Cause
Direct blow

Symptoms
Pain

Grating feeling in nose

Signs
Swelling

Discoloration

Possibly a deformity

Possibly bleeding

Inability to breathe through the nose

First Aid
Apply ice.

With your thumb and finger, gently pinch the nostrils shut with gauze if necessary to stop the bleeding.

Have the athlete sit with the head forward.

Send the athlete to a physician.

Playing Status
The athlete cannot return to activity until he or she is released by a physician.

The athlete should wear a nose protector when he or she returns to activity.

Prevention
Make sure athletes wear protective face masks and shields in football, lacrosse, and ice hockey.

Bloody Nose

Definition
This is a bleeding injury to the nose.

Causes
Direct blow to the nose

Possibly a head injury

High blood pressure

Dry nasal passages

Symptom
Pain if the athlete suffered from a direct blow

Signs
Bleeding nose

Possibly deformity or other signs of injury

First Aid
Have the athlete sit with the head forward.

Clamp the nostrils shut with your fingers to apply direct pressure, as in Figure 13.4.

You can apply ice to the bridge of the nose if the bleeding won't stop.

Send the athlete to a physician if the bleeding doesn't stop or if it was caused by another injury.

Do not let the athlete blow his or her nose.

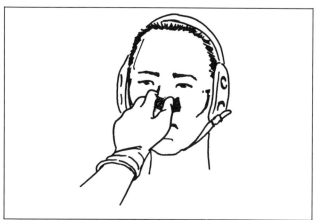

Figure 13.4   Bloody nose.

Playing Status
The athlete can return to activity once the bleeding stops for 5 minutes.

If the bleeding was caused by a more serious injury, the athlete must be released by a physician before returning to activity.

Prevention
Make sure athletes wear protective face masks and guards for football, ice hockey, and lacrosse.

Jaw Injury

Definition
A lower jaw injury may cause pain or popping when the athlete opens and closes the mouth or bites down. Fractures, contusions, and dislocations are the most common types of jaw injury.

Causes
Torsion injury or a direct blow to the jaw

Symptoms
Pain

The athlete complains of popping when he or she opens and closes the mouth.

Signs
Possibly deformity

Possibly discoloration

Swelling

Possibly an inability to close the mouth

The jaw may be out of place.

First Aid
Have the athlete rest.

Have the athlete sit with the head forward to allow blood and fluid to drain from the mouth.

Apply ice.

Send the athlete to a physician.

Playing Status
The athlete cannot return to activity until he or she is released by a physician.

Prevention
Make sure athletes wear helmets, mouth guards, and face masks when appropriate.

Chipped Tooth

Definition
This is a crack or break in a portion of a tooth (see Figure 13.5).

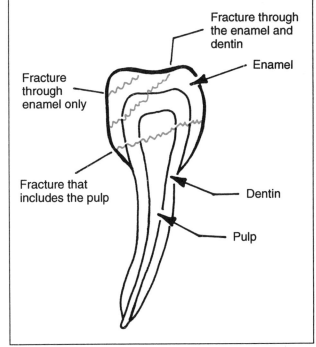

Figure 13.5 Chipped tooth.

Cause
Direct blow

History
The athlete was hit in the mouth with an object.

Symptoms
Possibly pain if the tooth is chipped down to the dentin or pulp

Possibly sensitivity to heat, cold, or pressure if the tooth is broken down to the dentin or pulp

Signs
Part of the tooth missing

Bleeding

Visible crack in a tooth

First Aid
Have the athlete sit with the head forward to allow blood to drain from the mouth.

Apply pressure with sterile gauze to any areas of the mouth that may be bleeding.

Send the athlete to a dentist as quickly as possible.

Playing Status
The athlete can return to activity after he or she is treated or is pain-free.

Prevention
Require athletes in contact sports to wear mouth guards.

Tooth Avulsion or Dislocated Tooth

Definition
The tooth is knocked out of its socket.

Cause
Direct blow

Symptom
Pain

Signs
Bleeding

Tooth totally dislodged

Swelling of the gums

First Aid
Immediately place the tooth in a container of milk or saline (contact lens) solution. If neither of these is available, use cold water as a substitute. Or, have the athlete hold the tooth in his or her mouth.

Place wet gauze over the socket and have the athlete bite down on it.

Have the athlete sit with the head forward to allow blood to drain from the mouth.

Transport the athlete to a dentist immediately! The tooth might be replaced successfully if done within an hour.

Playing Status
The athlete cannot return to activity until he or she is released by a dentist or oral surgeon.

Prevention
Require all athletes in contact sports to wear mouth guards.

Sport First Aid Recap

1. Cuts to the face and head often bleed heavily because the facial skin has an extensive network of blood vessels.

2. Most facial injuries are caused by a direct blow.

3. The most common eye injuries are contusions and lacerations.

4. When an eye contusion (black eye) occurs, always check for possible skull or eye damage.

5. Never try to remove a contact lens or embedded object from a lacerated eye. And bandage both eyes to protect the lacerated eye.

6. You can prevent the vast majority of ear avulsions by forbidding athletes to wear earrings during activity.

7. You can prevent most cases of cauliflower ear by requiring athletes to wear appropriate protective headgear during practices and games.

8. For broken noses and nosebleeds, apply gentle pressure by pinching the nostrils shut to help stop any bleeding.

9. Always have an athlete with a nosebleed lean forward, not back.

10. If the lower jaw is injured, the athlete will have pain and difficulty in biting down.

11. An athlete with a chipped or avulsed tooth should be taken immediately to a dentist or oral surgeon. An avulsed tooth must be saved and brought with the athlete to the dentist or surgeon.

CHAPTER 14

Skin Problems

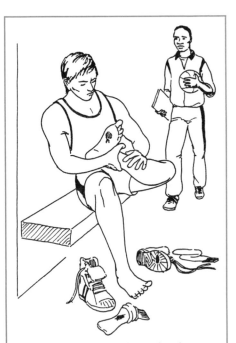

Dennis Bowles sits wincing with pain as he removes his sock in the locker room. He has just finished a hard preseason workout with the basketball team, and his feet are in bad shape. As he expects, the blister that has formed on the bottom of his left foot is bleeding. While Dennis is inspecting the sore, Coach Rick Holding walks by and spots the young athlete's injury. What should the coach do?

Skin injuries seem like such trivial problems, but are they really? Think about it. Did you ever have a nagging blister, scrape, or rash? It might have been only slightly uncomfortable to start with, but it probably bothered you a lot after a while, and especially when playing sports. If that was the case, it probably hurt your concentration and ultimately your performance. Not only that, but if handled improperly, skin injuries can lead to serious infections.

Your first aid goal for skin problems should be to prevent your athletes from being sidelined or distracted by these seemingly minor problems. The remainder of this chapter will describe the most common skin problems that you may see and tell you what you can do to stop them.

Callus

Definition
This is a buildup of rough skin that most often develops on the palm side of the hand, the sole of the foot, and the back of the heel. Although not a problem in themselves, calluses can lead to serious blisters.

Cause
Repeated friction or rubbing

Symptom
Feeling of roughness

Sign
Thick buildup of skin

First Aid
The athlete can file down calluses to prevent excessive skin buildup.

The athlete can also apply petroleum jelly over the spot to reduce friction.

Do not use a razor blade to remove a callus.

Prevention

It's best not to prevent small calluses because they help to protect vulnerable areas of the skin that are subjected to friction.

Have athletes use a file to keep calluses from accumulating too much buildup.

Blisters

Definition

A fluid-filled pocket arises between layers of the skin.

There are two types of blisters: open (see Figure 14.1) and closed.

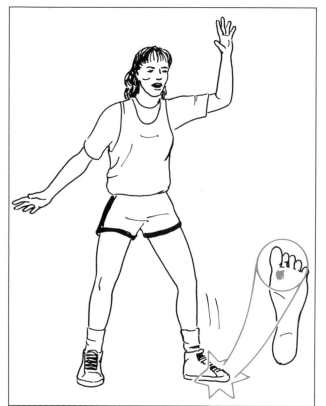

Figure 14.1 Open blister.

Cause

There is friction when the skin rubs against a surface such as a shoe, bat, or racket handle. The friction causes the skin layers to separate and fill with fluid.

Symptoms

Pain

Burning

Signs

Closed:

Fluid-filled bumps on skin

Open:

Possibly an open wound or bleeding

Redness around the area

Area may feel warm

First Aid

For Closed Blisters:

Tape a foam-rubber donut over the blister to reduce friction, as shown in Figure 14.2.

Have the athlete keep the area clean and rub the blistered area with an ice cube.

Do not open the blister, or it may become infected.

For Open Blisters:

Clean the area with antiseptic soap, alcohol, or peroxide.

Dry the area with a sterile gauze pad.

Tape a foam rubber donut over the blister to reduce friction.

Have the athlete keep the area clean.

Periodically check the area for signs of infection.

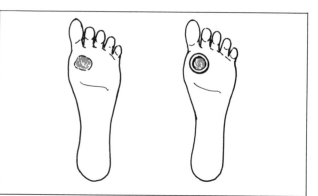

Figure 14.2 Protective donut pad for blisters.

Prevention

Have athletes file calluses to prevent excessive skin buildup.

Have athletes apply ice over skin hot spots (reddened areas that have not yet formed blisters).

Have athletes apply petroleum jelly to reduce friction over vulnerable areas.

Make sure athletes protect their hands with gloves in sports such as racquetball, baseball, weight lifting, and golf.

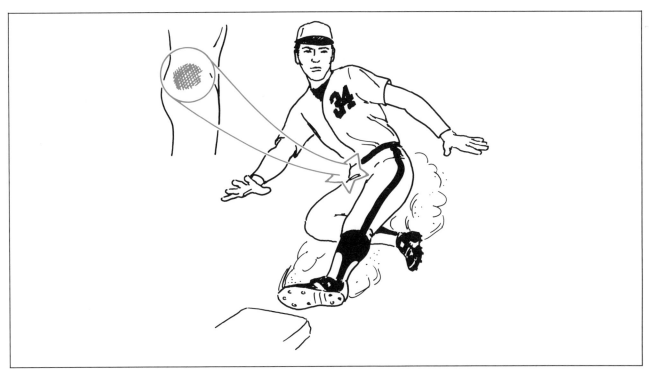

Figure 14.3 Abrasion.

Abrasion

Definition
This is a scraping injury to the superficial layer of skin (see Figure 14.3) (also known as turf burns and strawberries).

Cause
Sliding or falling against a rough or hard surface

Symptoms
Pain

Tight or pulling feeling of skin (scab) over healing abrasions

Burning sensation

Sign
Red patch of skin

First Aid
Clean with antiseptic soap, alcohol, or peroxide.

During activity, moisten the area with petroleum jelly or cover with a sterile gauze pad.

Prevention
Make sure athletes wear sliding pants or protective padding over the elbows, knees, and hips.

Athlete's Foot

Definition
This is a contagious fungal infection of the skin on the feet.

Cause
Allowing feet to stay sweaty, hot, and covered, which promotes fungal growth

Symptoms
Burning

Itching

Sign
Red, scaly rash around the toes and other areas of the feet

First Aid
Make sure the athlete keeps the feet dry and warm by changing socks frequently.

Have the athletes use foot powder to absorb sweat.

Have the athlete apply antifungal cream or powder to the area.

Send the athlete to a physician if the symptoms persist.

Prevention
Encourage athletes to keep their feet clean and dry.

Make sure athletes always wear clean socks.

Have athletes protect their feet in the locker room and shower by wearing thongs.

Jock Itch

Definition
This is a fungal infection affecting the groin area.

Cause
Sweaty, hot area promotes fungal growth

Symptoms
Burning pain in the genital area

Itching in the genital area

Sign
Red, scaly patches of skin

First Aid
Instruct the athlete to keep the area dry by changing wet, sweaty clothing.

Have the athlete use powder to help absorb sweat.

Have the athlete apply antifungal powder or cream to the infected area.

Send the athlete to a physician if symptoms persist.

Prevention
Have athletes use powder to help absorb sweat.

Recommend that athletes wear clean workout clothes daily.

Burns

Definition
Skin cells are destroyed by coming in contact with or being exposed to very hot surfaces, sun, or fire.

Cause
The most common causes in sport are sunburn and chemical burns from leaking commercial cold packs.

Symptoms
Burning or stinging pain felt over the affected area

The athlete complains of skin feeling hot.

Signs
Redness

Swelling

Blisters, in severe cases

Area feels hot

First Aid
Keep the area clean and dry.

Do not wash or apply ointment to open wounds; instead, apply a sterile dressing.

Flush chemical burns with cool water for several minutes.

Send an athlete with an infected or extensive burn to a physician.

Prevention
Require athletes to wear sunscreen while participating outdoors.

Use crushed-ice packs instead of commercial cold packs.

Boils

Definition
These are large, infected, pus-filled bumps on the skin.

Cause
Athletes who have a low stress tolerance are prone to boils.

Symptom
The athlete complains of a painful bump on the skin.

Signs
Red and possibly white bump on the skin

Area may feel warm

First Aid
Apply ice over the area to help decrease the pain and swelling.

Send the athlete to a physician.

Do not puncture the boil.

Prevention
Encourage athletes to get plenty of rest and eat a balanced diet.

Poison Ivy

Definition
This uncomfortable skin reaction is caused by contact with poison ivy plants.

Cause
Contact with poison ivy—plants, vines, or shrubs like those shown in Figure 14.4.

Symptoms
Burning over the affected area

Itching

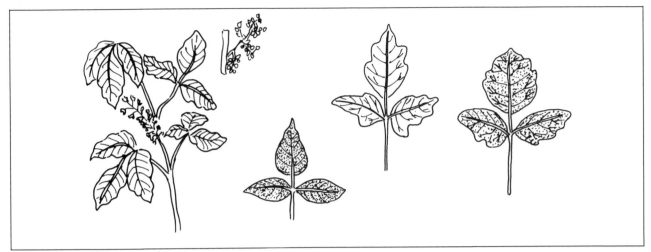

Figure 14.4 Common poison ivy.

Signs
Redness

Rash

Swelling

Blisters

High fever, if condition worsens

First Aid
Remove all contaminated clothing.

Clean the area with soap and water.

Send the athlete to a physician.

Warn the athlete not to scratch the area.

Prevention
Clear the playing area of poison ivy.

Educate athletes about poison ivy, and warn them to stay away from infested areas.

Sport First Aid Recap

1. By acting quickly and appropriately, you can prevent skin problems from sidelining your athletes.

2. Keep all wound areas clean to prevent infection.

3. Never attempt to open blisters or boils.

4. Protect injured areas from further harm by applying sterile gauze or foam rubber.

5. If symptoms persist or if the athlete develops an infection, the athlete should be sent to a physician.

APPENDIX A

The American Sport Education Program and the National Federation Interscholastic Coaches Education Program

History

The American Coaching Effectiveness Program (ACEP) began in 1976 when Dr. Rainer Martens, then a professor at the University of Illinois, launched it through the university's Office of Youth Sports. The effort involved examining coaching education programs, surveying coaches, consulting national sport agencies, and synthesizing research in the sport sciences. The first version of the ACEP curriculum was released in 1981, focusing on youth sport. Instructors originally conducted the clinics using a slide-and-lecture format.

When feedback indicated the need for easier presentation, ACEP updated its initial course, releasing an instructional video in January 1987. This second edition of the ACEP Level 1 curriculum proved popular, and more and more high school and national organization administrators turned to ACEP for help in adequately preparing their coaches.

Since then, we have been continually work-ing to improve the quality and scope of our offerings. In 1990 the National Federation of State High School Associations (NFSHSA) selected ACEP as the official education program for the National Federation Interscholastic Coaches Association (NFICA). A special version of ACEP's Leader Level curriculum was released as the National Federation Interscholastic Coaches Education Program (NFICEP), improving further the quality of coaching throughout the United States. To meet the needs of coaches for education in providing an initial emergency response to injured athletes, the ACEP/NFICEP collaboration soon added a Sport First Aid Course, and ACEP continued to expand its program offerings to meet coaches' wide ranging needs.

In 1994, ACEP expanded its mission beyond coaching education, to include programs for parents and sport administrators. Accordingly, ACEP became the American Sport Education Program (ASEP). ASEP and NFSHSA continued to work together, and in the summer of 1996, we released a new course, the Drugs and

163

Sport Course. This course was developed in response to the growing need among coaches and sport administrators to help bring effective prevention messages to our nation's athletes.

This publication marks still further collaboration between ASEP and NFSHSA. The original ASEP and NFICEP coaching course is now the Coaching Principles Course (the recently updated second edition of *Successful Coaching* serves as the course text), and this updated edition of *Sport First Aid* represents revision of the Sport First Aid Course. Both these updated courses reflect the latest in sport science and sports medicine, helping ASEP and NFSHSA to provide state-of-the-art education for coaches.

NFICA

The National Federation Interscholastic Coaches Association (NFICA), formed in 1981 as a professional organization of the National Federation of State High School Associations, now serves some 40,000 members. A small annual membership fee brings many benefits, including liability insurance, opportunities to serve on rules committees, and a subscription to the National Federation Coaches' Quarterly—a new publication designed specifically for high school coaches. NFICA affords impor-

tant leadership involvement to its state coaches associations and holds an annual spring leadership conference to help coaches develop able state leaders.

ASEP Curriculum

ASEP's mission has always been to provide safe, meaningful, and enjoyable sport experiences for athletes by educating coaches in the areas of coaching philosophy, sport science, sports medicine, and sport techniques and tactics. Sport administrators and parents also play vital roles in shaping sport experiences, and ASEP's curriculum is designed to provide educational resources for all these key players—coaches, parents, sport administrators, and soon, officials—to help them better fulfill their roles.

ASEP's curriculum is available to coaches, administrators, and parents for programs involving youth, interscholastic, and club sport and beyond. This multilevel curriculum is presented in the chart on page 165.

For up-to-date information on the availability and prices of curricular and other resources, call the ASEP National Center at 800-747-5698, write to us at P.O. Box 5076, Champaign, IL, 61825-5076, or e-mail us at asep@hkusa.com. You may also visit ASEP on the World Wide Web at http://www.asep.com/.

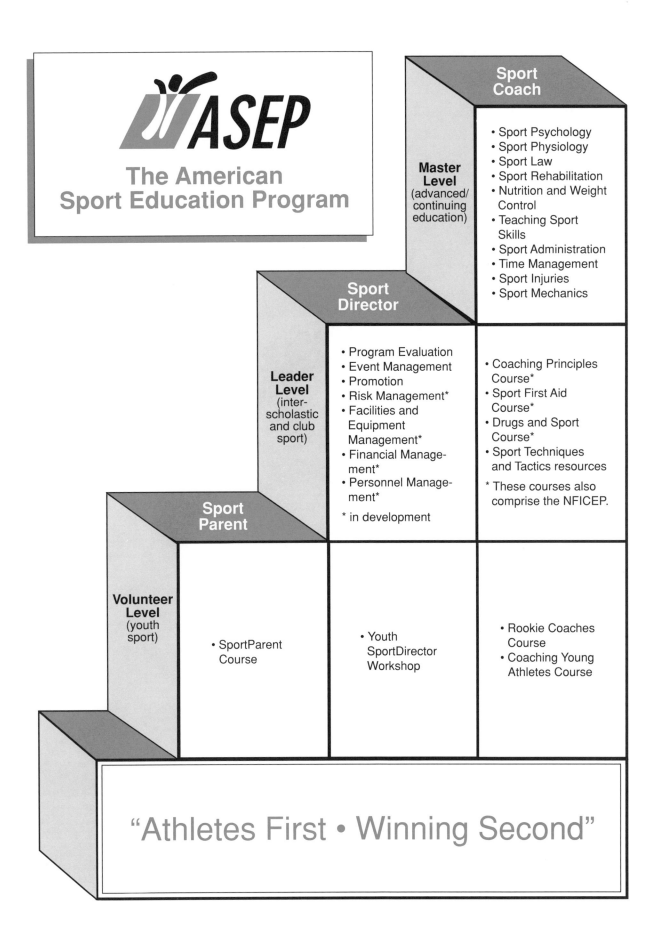

ASEP
The American
Sport Education Program

Sport Coach

Master Level (advanced/ continuing education)

- Sport Psychology
- Sport Physiology
- Sport Law
- Sport Rehabilitation
- Nutrition and Weight Control
- Teaching Sport Skills
- Sport Administration
- Time Management
- Sport Injuries
- Sport Mechanics

Sport Director

Leader Level (inter-scholastic and club sport)

- Program Evaluation
- Event Management
- Promotion
- Risk Management*
- Facilities and Equipment Management*
- Financial Management*
- Personnel Management*

* in development

- Coaching Principles Course*
- Sport First Aid Course*
- Drugs and Sport Course*
- Sport Techniques and Tactics resources

* These courses also comprise the NFICEP.

Sport Parent

Volunteer Level (youth sport)

- SportParent Course

- Youth SportDirector Workshop

- Rookie Coaches Course
- Coaching Young Athletes Course

"Athletes First • Winning Second"

APPENDIX B

Injury-Prevention Stretching Routine

Technique—Stretch to the point of a gentle pull, then hold 10 counts without bouncing. Perform at least 10 repetitions 5 days a week.

Warm-up—Do 5 to 10 minutes of low-intensity aerobic activity such as jogging, walking, or calisthenics. Then perform two repetitions of each stretch.

Cool-down—Walk around to allow the heart and breathing rates to return to normal. Then perform 6 to 8 repetitions of each stretch before the muscles cool.

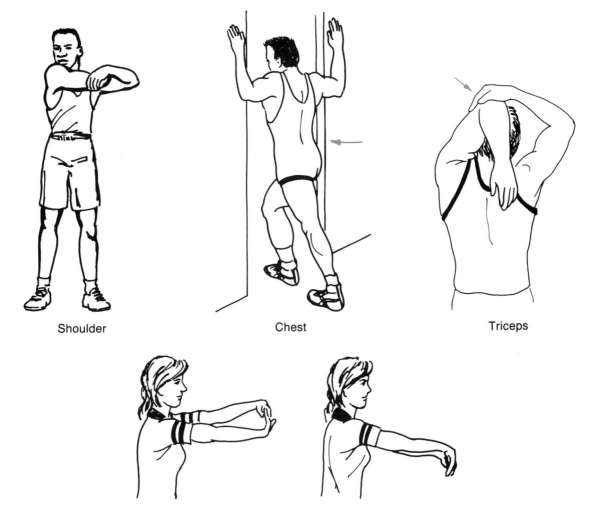

Shoulder   Chest   Triceps

Elbow and forearm

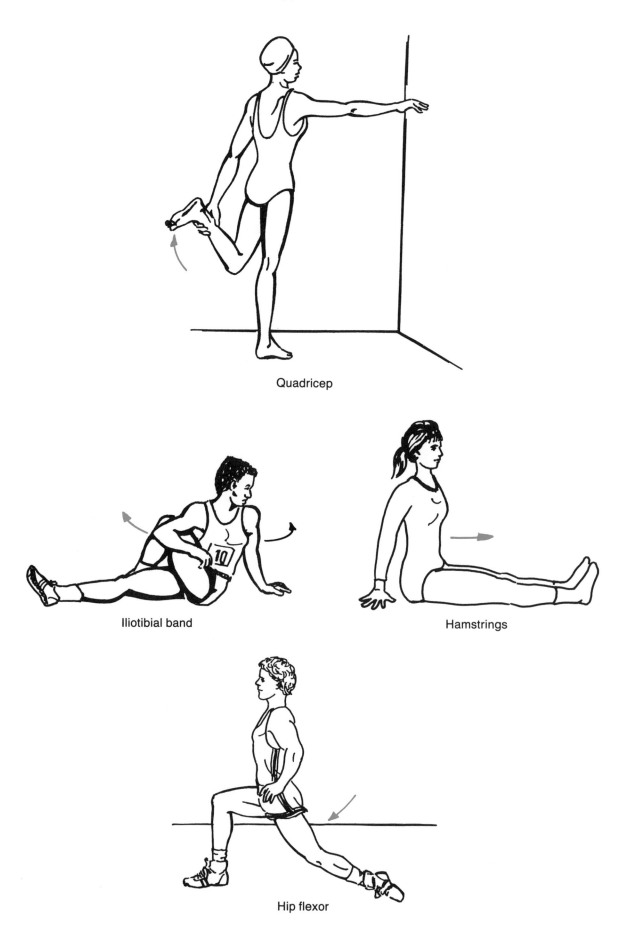

Quadricep

Iliotibial band

Hamstrings

Hip flexor

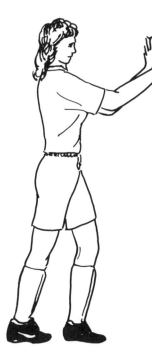 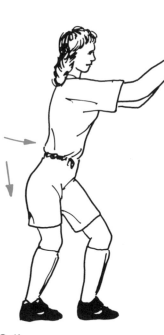

Calf

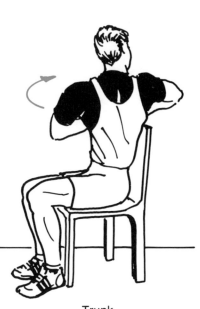

Trunk

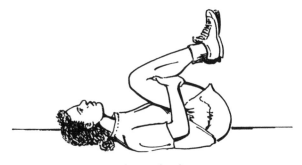

Lower back

Important Sport First Aid Terms

ABCs—Acronym for monitoring the airway, breathing, and circulation of an injury victim.

abrasion—Scraping injury. Examples: turf burns, strawberries.

Achilles tendon—Tendon attaching the calf muscles to the heel bone.

acute—Occurring suddenly. Examples: fractures and sprains.

airway—Passage through which air travels to the lungs. Includes the nose, mouth, and windpipe (trachea).

alveoli—Air sacs where oxygen and carbon dioxide are exchanged by the capillaries in the lungs.

anaphylactic shock—Life-threatening allergic reaction that can cause the air passages to close. Commonly happens as the result of bee stings.

artery—Large blood vessel that carries oxygen to the tissues.

asthma—Condition in which the air passages in the lungs constrict and interfere with normal breathing.

athlete's foot—Fungal infection to the foot caused by exposure to a moist, warm environment.

avulsion—Forceful tearing of a structure, especially the bones or skin.

blister—Fluid-filled bump between skin layers. Caused by friction between layers.

boil—Large infected bump on the skin.

brachial artery—Major artery supplying oxygen-carrying blood to the arm.

bronchial tubes—Tubes through which air passes through to the lungs.

burner—Pinched nerve in the neck or shoulder.

bursa—Fluid-filled sacs located in the joints. Help to reduce friction between tendons, bones, and other joint structures.

bursitis—Inflammation of the bursa, which causes it to swell and become warm.

callus—Skin buildup over areas of friction, especially on the palm of the hands, the heels, or the feet.

capillaries—Smallest blood vessel that aids in the exchange of oxygen and carbon dioxide between blood and tissue cells.

cardiac arrest—When heart stops beating.

cardiopulmonary resuscitation (CPR)—First aid for cardiac and respiratory arrest.

carotid pulse—Heartbeat felt at the carotid artery in the neck.

cartilage—Gristlelike connective tissue usually found covering ends of bones. It protects the bones from friction and shock.

cauliflower ear—Contusion to the outside ear.

171

cervical spine—Neck portion of the spinal column.

chronic—Prolonged or gradually occurring.

circulatory system—System that supplies blood to the body. Includes the heart, arteries, arterioles, veins, and capillaries, as well as other structures.

closed fracture—Broken bone that does not break through the skin.

compression—Application of pressure over an area to reduce bleeding or swelling.

concussion—Temporary malfunction of the brain resulting from a direct blow to the head. Can cause memory loss, dizziness, headache, nausea, unconsciousness, etc.

contusion—Bruising injury causing bleeding, swelling, and discoloration.

convulsion—Seizure; violent muscle contractions.

dehydration—Low level of water in the body.

diabetes—Disorder in which the body is unable to produce or regulate the insulin needed to control blood sugar levels.

diabetic coma—Condition in which the body's blood sugar levels rise too high. Also known as hyperglycemia.

diabetic shock—Condition in which the body's blood sugar levels drop too low. Also known as hypoglycemia. Causes dizziness, confusion, cool and clammy skin, etc.

digestive system—System that breaks food down into substances that can be used as fuel by the body tissues.

direct pressure—Application of pressure over a wound to help stop bleeding.

elevation—Raising of a body part above heart level.

epiphyseal fracture—Growth plate fracture.

extension—Straightening of a joint.

fainting—Temporary loss of consciousness; a mild form of shock.

femoral artery—Major blood vessel carrying oxygen-filled blood to the leg.

flexion—Bending of a joint.

fracture—Break in a bone.

frostbite—Freezing of the superficial skin tissues and possibly deeper tissues such as muscles.

glucose—Form of sugar used by the body for energy.

growth plate—Area on the ends of bones where growth takes place.

hamstrings—Muscles located on the back of the thigh. Help to bend the knee and extend the hip.

heat cramps—Muscle cramps caused by dehydration or loss of electrolytes through sweat.

heat exhaustion—Shocklike condition caused by dehydration. A key sign of heat exhaustion is profuse sweating. Other signs include cool and clammy skin.

heatstroke—Life-threatening illness caused by extreme dehydration. Body temperature rises to 105 degrees or higher and the skin is red, hot, and dry.

Heimlich maneuver—First aid for choking.

hip pointer—Contusion or bruise to the pelvic bone located on the front of the hip.

history—Information gathered to help determine the nature, extent, and mechanism of an injury.

hyperextension—Straightening of a joint past its normal range.

hyperflexion—bending of a joint beyond its normal bending range.

hyperglycemia—High blood sugar level, often caused by diabetes.

hypoglycemia—Low blood sugar level, often caused by diabetes.

hypothermia—Condition in which the body temperature lowers to abnormally low levels. Caused by extreme fatigue and exposure to a cold, windy environment.

impingement—Injury in which tissue is pinched between two surfaces.

incision—Soft-tissue cut caused by a sharp object.

inflammation—Irritation to a body structure. Often causes swelling, scar tissue, and heat in the area.

inspection—Evaluation technique used to determine the nature of an injury. Inspection signs to look for include swelling, discoloration, deformity, skin color, etc.

insulin—Hormone or chemical that enables body tissues to use sugar or glucose as energy.

inversion—injury in which the ankle is twisted inward.

jock itch—Fungal infection of the genital area.

joint—Junction between bones that allows the body to move. Examples: knee, elbow, shoulder, ankle, and wrist.

kidney—Organ of the urinary system used to help rid the body of energy breakdown waste products.

laceration—Soft-tissue cut caused by a blow with a blunt object.

ligament—Fibrous tissue that connects bone to bone and prevents bones from shifting over each other. Primary stabilizers of the body joints.

loss of function—Inability of a body part to carry out its function because of injury. Example: Loss of function at the knee would be an inability to bend or straighten it.

lumbar spine—Portion of the spinal column located at the low back area.

lungs—Organs in which oxygen and carbon dioxide are exchanged between the air and the capillaries.

mechanism of injury—Cause of an injury; may be sudden or gradual. Examples: direct blow, twisting, or friction injuries.

open fracture—Broken bone that pierces the skin.

orthopedist—Physician who specializes in caring for musculoskeletal injuries and disorders.

Osgood-Schlatter disease—Irritation to the junction where the kneecap tendon inserts into the lower leg bone.

overuse—Injury caused by overusing a weak or inflexible muscle, tendon, or bone. Can cause the tissue to gradually swell, become painful, and lose function.

patella—Kneecap.

podiatrist—Doctor who specializes in handling disorders of the legs and feet.

pressure points—Areas where pressure should be applied to reduce blood flow to an area. Located in the upper arm and leg. Used as a last resort in controlling bleeding in the arms or legs.

PRICE—Protection, rest, ice, compression, and elevation.

primary survey—Inspection of the ABCs, or airway, breathing, and circulation, to determine possible problems.

puncture—Deep, narrow soft-tissue wound caused by being stabbed with a thin object.

quadriceps—Muscle located on the front of the thigh. It helps to straighten the knee and move the thigh forward.

radial pulse—Heartbeat felt at the wrist.

rescue breathing—First aid for respiratory arrest.

respiratory arrest—When breathing stops.

respiratory system—System that exchanges oxygen and carbon dioxide between the air and the blood. Includes the nose, mouth, windpipe, and lungs.

rotator cuff—Group of four muscles located on the shoulder blade. They are used primarily in throwing and overhead shoulder motions, as well as in forehand and backhand strokes.

secondary survey—Inspection conducted after the primary survey to determine the site, location, and severity of other injuries. Includes HIT, or history, inspection, and touch.

seizures—Violent muscle spasms or convulsions.

shearing—Injury involving friction or rubbing between two surfaces.

shinsplints—Overuse injury to the lower leg often caused by muscle weakness and inflexibility.

shock—Systemic body reaction to physical or emotional injury. The body deprives the skin, arms, legs, and other less essential tissues of oxygen and blood to ensure supplies to the brain, heart, and lungs.

side stitch—Pain in the side felt during endurance activities.

sign—Physical evidence of injury. Includes swelling, discoloration, deformity, etc.

solar plexus—Nervous system structure that assists in breathing. Located near the stomach.

sprain—Stretch or tear of a ligament.

strain—Stretch or tear of a muscle or tendon.

stress fracture—Bone fracture caused by overuse. The fracture develops slowly while the bone is experiencing repeated stress such as in long-distance running.

sweating—Mechanism through which the body cools itself. Water is transported to the skin, where it is evaporated to cool the body.

symptoms—Complaint(s) associated with injury. Includes pain, numbness, tingling, and grating feelings.

tendinitis—Inflammation of a tendon. Causes swelling, warmth, and scar tissue.

tendon—Fibroelastic structure that connects muscle to bone.

tennis elbow—Inflammation of the junction where the wrist and forearm muscles attach to the outside of the upper arm bone.

thoracic spine—Portion of the spinal column located at the upper and midback area.

torsion—Twisting injury.

trachea—Passage in the neck through which air passes from the mouth to the bronchial tubes. Also known as the windpipe.

vertebrae—Bones of the spinal column.

vital signs—ABCs, or breathing and heart rates.

windchill—Index used to indicate the effect of wind on cold temperatures.

Recommended Readings

Books

Arnheim, D. (1984). *Modern principles of athletic training*. St. Louis: C.V. Mosby.

Bergeron, J.D., & Greene, H.W. (1989). *Coaches guide to sport injuries*. Champaign, IL: Human Kinetics.

Booher, J.M., & Thibodeau, G.A. (Eds.) (1989). *Athletic injury assessment* (2nd ed.). St. Louis: C.V. Mosby.

Eisenman, P.A., Johnson, S.C., & Benson, J.E. (1990). *Coaches guide to nutrition and weight control* (2nd ed.). Champaign, IL: Leisure Press.

Fahey, T.D. (1986). *Athletic training: Principles and practices*. Mountain View, CA: Mayfield.

Guten, G.N. (1991). *Play healthy, stay healthy: Your guide to managing and treating 40 common sports injuries*. Champaign, IL: Human Kinetics.

Micheli, L. (1995). *The sports medicine bible*. New York: Perennial.

Roy, S.P., & Irvin, R.F. (1983). *Sports medicine: Prevention, evaluation, management, and rehabilitation*. Englewood Cliffs, NJ: Prentice Hall.

Steele, M.K. (1996). *Sideline help: A guide for immediate evaluation and care for sports injuries*. Champaign, IL: Human Kinetics.

Tippett, S.R. (1990). *Coaches guide to sport rehabilitation*. Champaign, IL: Leisure Press.

Journals

Athletic Therapy Today (Champaign, IL: Human Kinetics).

Athletic Training (Dallas: National Athletic Trainers Association)

The First Aider (Gardner, KS: Cramer Products)

Physician & Sportsmedicine (Minneapolis: McGraw-Hill)

References

Curtis, N. (1996). Job outlook for athletic trainers. *Athletic Therapy Today*, **1**(2), 7-11.

Eisenman, P.A., Johnson, S.C., & Benson, J.E. (1990). *Coaches guide to nutrition and weight control.* 2nd ed. Champaign, IL: Human Kinetics.

Legwold, G. (1983). Injury rate lowered by high school trainer. *Physician & Sportsmedicine*, **12**, 35-36.

Martens, R.M. (1997). *Successful coaching.* Updated 2nd ed. Champaign, IL: Human Kinetics.

National Athletic Trainers Association. (1989a). Public relations: 3-year study finds 'major injuries' up 20% in high school football. *Athletic Training*, **24**, 60-69.

National Athletic Trainers Association. (1989b). Public relations: Injury toll in prep sports estimated at 1.3 million. *Athletic Training*, **24**, 360-367.

Nygaard, G., & Boone, T.H. (1985). *Coaches guide to sport law.* Champaign, IL: Human Kinetics.

Rice, S.G. (1995). Sports injuries studied for 13 years at 20 high schools in Washington. *National Federation News*, **13**(3), 9-11.

Rowe, P.J., & Robertson, D.M. (1986). Knowledge of care and prevention of athletic injuries in high schools. *Athletic Training*, **21**, 116-119.

Sharkey, B. (1986). *Coaches guide to sport physiology.* Champaign, IL: Human Kinetics.

Weidner, T.G. (1989). Injuries—Are coaches prepared? *Journal of Physical Education, Recreation, and Dance*, **60**, 82-84.

Welch, T.F. (1996). NATA releases results from high school injury study. *NATA News*, April, 16-23.

Index

Page numbers in **bold** type indicate figures and illustrations

About the Author

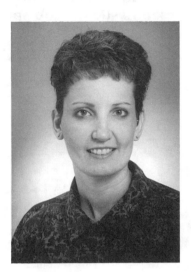

Providing first aid for injured athletes is a daily activity for Melinda Flegel. She is head athletic trainer at the University of Illinois SportWell Center, where her responsibilities include overseeing sports medicine care for the university's recreational and club sport athletes as well as providing them with educational and preventive programs.

As coordinator of outreach services at the Great Plains Sports Medicine and Rehabilitation Center in Peoria, Illinois, Flegel annually assisted coaches at some 15 schools in providing first aid for their athletes. Her roles as the center's educational program coordinator and American Red Cross CPR instructor gave her firsthand experience in helping coaches become proficient first responders.

Flegel, a certified athletic trainer, received a master's degree in physical education from the University of Illinois in 1982. A member of the National Athletic Trainers Association, she has been a reviewer for the association's journal, *Athletic Training*, and a member of the Illinois Athletic Trainers Association Clinic and Industrial Trainers Committee. She is also a certified strength and conditioning specialist through the National Strength and Conditioning Association. In her leisure time, Flegel plays volleyball, squash, and softball and enjoys photography and drawing.

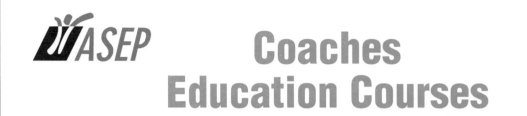

ASEP

Coaches Education Courses

NFICEP/ASEP Leader Level provides the following training courses and resources for coaches and administrators in interscholastic or club sport:

Sport First Aid Coaches Course

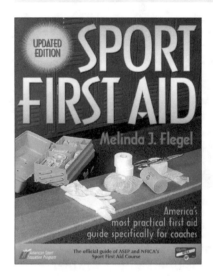

The Sport First Aid Course consists of a 4-hour clinic based on this updated first edition of *Sport First Aid*. After the clinic, coaches study this text and take an open-book test.

Sport First Aid Course Package

(Consists of *Sport First Aid* (Updated Edition), clinic study guide, and test packet and processing)

Item ACEP0096 • $35.00 per coach

The Sport First Aid Course teaches coaches how to develop a plan for emergency procedures, prevent avoidable injuries, evaluate serious and minor injuries, provide proper, immediate care for common problems, and respond to life-threatening emergencies.

Drugs and Sport Coaches Course

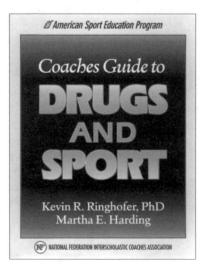

This course, based on the text *Coaches Guide to Drugs and Sport*, consists of a 4-hour clinic. After the clinic, coaches study the text and take an open-book test.

(Consists of *Coaches Guide to Drugs and Sport*, clinic study guide, and test packet and processing)

Item ACEP0093 • $35.00 per coach

The Drugs and Sport Course teaches coaches how to recognize and capitalize on their positions as role models; communicate effective tobacco, alcohol, and other drug use prevention messages; and respond to athletes who exhibit symptoms of concern.

Coaching Principles Coaches Course

This course, based on the text *Successful Coaching* (Updated Second Edition), consists of a 7-hour clinic. After the clinic, coaches study the text and take an open-book test.

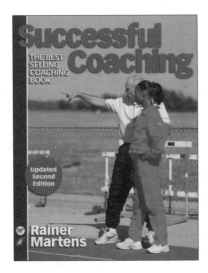

Coaching Principles Course Package

(Consists of *Successful Coaching*, clinic study guide, and test packet and processing)

Item ACEP0120 • $35.00 per coach

This course is excellent for both new and experienced coaches with little formal coaching education. It combines the practical expertise of veteran coaches with the important new findings of sport scientists.

The Coaching Principles Course teaches coaches how to

- ✓ keep winning in perspective,
- ✓ develop a functional coaching philosophy,
- ✓ communicate well with their athletes,
- ✓ motivate athletes,
- ✓ teach skills effectively,
- ✓ develop a physical training program,
- ✓ guide athletes to better nutrition,
- ✓ reduce injuries by managing risks better, and
- ✓ manage equipment, facilities, schedules, and other team logistics effectively.

For more information on NFICEP or ASEP's Leader Level, call Toll-Free, fax, write, or visit our Web site.

About NFICEP and ASEP's Leader Level

The National Federation Interscholastic Coaches Education Program (NFICEP) is the coaching education program of the National Federation of State High School Associations and is endorsed by interscholastic organizations in 40 states. NFICEP is a special version of the American Sport Education Program (ASEP) Leader Level SportCoach Program.

ASEP, the nation's leader in coaching education since 1981, has provided education for more than 700,000 coaches, parents, and sport administrators through its multilevel curriculum.

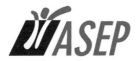

American Sport Education Program
P.O. Box 5076
Champaign, IL 61825-5076
Toll-Free 1-800-747-5698
Fax: 217-351-1549
http://www.asep.com/